FLORENCE NIGHTINGALE

THE WOUNDED SOLDIER'S FRIEND

By

ELIZA F. POLLARD

WITH A CHAPTER FROM
Reminiscences of Linda Richards
BY LINDA RICHARDS

First published in 1891

Copyright © 2020 Brilliant Women

This edition is published by Brilliant Women,
an imprint of Read & Co.

This book is copyright and may not be reproduced or copied in any way without the express permission of the publisher in writing.

British Library Cataloguing-in-Publication Data
A catalogue record for this book is available
from the British Library.

Read & Co. is part of Read Books Ltd.
For more information visit
www.readandcobooks.co.uk

The world's a room of sickness, where each heart
   Knows its own anguish and unrest;
The truest wisdom there, and noblest art,
   Is his, who skills of comfort best;
Whom by the softest step and gentlest tone
   Enfeebled spirits own,
And love to raise the languid eye,
When, like an angel's wing, they feel him fleeting by.

JOHN KEBLE

RECOLLECTIONS OF FLORENCE NIGHTINGALE

BY LINDA RICHARDS, AMERICA'S FIRST TRAINED NURSE

In May, 1877, through the influence of Miss Nightingale, I was invited to visit St. Thomas Hospital Training School for as long a time as I wished. I went to the School and was made most welcome and comfortable for two months. I was given every advantage for observation in everything concerning the school and gained much valuable knowledge. I had been in the school only a few days when Miss Nightingale invited me to call upon her in her home. I went and was taken by the maid to Miss Nightingale's room -- .a large square room in which was a bed so placed that one could go around it without touching it. Upon the bed, dressed in black silk with a pretty lace cap upon her head, was Miss Nightingale. What I noticed particularly was her beautifully shaped head and her clear blue eyes which looked straight into mine. She extended a small delicate hand which gave mine a very friendly grasp; a chair was placed for me by the side of her bed, and for one hour we talked all about our own and English hospitals and training schools. While I was there a dainty lunch was served me. Miss Nightingale took particular interest in my work in London, and Edinburgh, advising me regarding the best hospitals to visit, and through her influence I was admitted to King's College Hospital as a visitor and also to the Royal Infirmary of Edinburgh. She invited me to visit her at her country home in Lee Hurst, where I spent several most enjoyable days, seeing Miss Nightingale some time each day and gaining much from her in every way. She questioned me carefully concerning our methods and the making of our young schools, and when I left her she said, "May you outstrip us that we may in turn outstrip you." To have had the honour of meeting Miss Nightingale I esteem as one of my greatest blessings.

A Chapter from
Reminiscences of Linda Richards, 1911

PREFACE

*"Wearing the white flower of a blameless life
Before a thousand peering littlenesses."*

IN these pages I have attempted to write the life of one who has recently departed from amongst us, and whose death brought the memory of her vividly back to those who knew and loved her for the work she wrought whilst living. To the younger generation she is a familiar name—to them, "by her deeds she is known."

Comparatively few were admitted into the sacred precincts of her private life; only those who needed her help, who worked with or for her, or those who were linked to her by ties of blood and friendship, approached her.

Like all noble souls Florence Nightingale cared little for the praise of men, in the accomplishment of the work which she did for Christ's sake.

PREFACE.

I, a woman, am writing a woman's life, and shall strive to bring before those who read this book the lesson she taught, that "There is work to our hand," if we will but see it; work of the very highest order, —the caring for that "Temple," which is the "Temple" of the living God, the human body, which Christ took upon Himself, and thereby sanctified and honoured.

To write of one who was with us but a few years ago, whose living presence is, so to speak, still hovering over us, is no easy task, and yet the simple beauty of Florence Nightingale's life minimises the difficulty in her case—there is such tender austerity in her character. Like our Saviour's, her life's work was begun and ended in the space of three years, but the work she accomplished is, like His, immortal. At her country's call she left her beautiful home to succour and to help—as only she could do—the brave men who were dying for that country—hers and theirs! Her work done, she went home again. Since then her *voice* has been heard, her *spirit* has been felt, and will continue to be felt amongst us from generation to generation. She herself remained in the background, partly from ill health, but more especially because the work she had set herself to do lay in itself so near her heart, that any appearance of personal vanity, anything that might throw a slur upon it or call in question the purity of her motives, would have been pain and grief to her.

She had a lesson to teach, which she learnt first herself and then gave forth by precept and example

PREFACE.

to the world : the law of order and obedience, and the necessity of systematic training, by which alone knowledge and power can be acquired for the overcoming of vice and the bringing of help and relief to suffering humanity.

Christ went up to Jerusalem, and was found by His mother in the Temple in the midst of the Rabbis, "both hearing and asking them questions." Afterwards He went back with her to Nazareth, and bided His time ; but from that hour He was about " His Father's business." Even when in the workshop with Joseph He was in "training," preparing for those three short years of ministry which were to change the moral face of the whole earth.

This is the great lesson Florence Nightingale brought into evidence, that nursing the sick, and tending the poor, must be done systematically, with order ; not as desultory work to be taken up and dropped as the whim of the moment may dictate, but as a high and noble calling, worthy to be undertaken by the greatest lady in the land, even as by the humblest member of Christ's flock, if their hearts be in the work. Not for themselves must they labour, but for God ; that is the keynote of her teaching and of her work. Self must be put away ; not by acts of asceticism and mortification, but by the power of love—of Divine love.

For those who enter upon it in this spirit, we will quote her own words:—" I give a quarter of a century's European experience, when I say the happiest people, the fondest of their occupation, the most thankful for their lives, are, in my opinion, those engaged in sick

PREFACE.

nursing. It is a mere abuse of words to represent the life, as is done by some, as a sacrifice and martyrdom.

"In the natural course of events, there have been martyrs, in this as in every other great movement—the founders and pioneers of everything that is best and noblest, must be content to be martyrs. But they rarely think of themselves as such. There must be constant self-sacrifice in all things for the good of others. But a nurse's life, if rightly viewed, is not a life of sacrifice; it is engaging in an occupation the happiest of any. The strong, the healthy wills in any life, must determine to pursue the common good at any personal cost, at daily sacrifice; and we must not think that any fit of enthusiasm will carry us through such a life as this.

"Nothing but the feeling that it is God's work more than ours, that we are seeking *His* success not *our* success, and that we have trained and fitted ourselves by every means which He has granted us to carry out His work, will enable us to go on."

Florence Nightingale's whole teaching is, from first to last, summed up in these words, "Love of God and forgetfulness of self."

ELIZA F. POLLARD.

CONTENTS

I. EARLY DAYS 11

II. "AN EXAMPLE" 25

III. IN TRAINING 41

IV. "FOR QUEEN AND COUNTRY" 55

V. "THE CALL" 68

VI. "AT THE HELM" 82

VII. A MESSAGE 95

VIII. FAITHFUL UNTO DEATH 107

IX. A NATION'S GRATITUDE 123

X. ADIEU 132

XI. IN MEMORIAM 143

XII. HOME AT LAST! 152

FLORENCE NIGHTINGALE

THE WOUNDED SOLDER'S FRIEND

CHAPTER I.

EARLY DAYS.

> "Little efforts work great actions;
> Lessons in our childhood taught
> Mould the spirit of that temper
> Wherein mighty deeds are wrought.
>
> "Cherish then the gifts of childhood,
> Use them gently, guard them well;
> For their future growth and greatness
> Who can measure, who can tell?"
> Mrs. Alexander.

"LOOK at old Roger, what can have happened, his sheep are scattered all over the hill-side, and he is calling after them, but they don't seem to listen much?"

The speaker, a little girl of about ten years old, mounted on a shaggy pony, pointed with her whip to where a flock of sheep was running hither and thither regardless of the voice of an old shepherd, who, with his sheep-skin over his shoulders and his tall crook in his hand, was vainly striving to keep them together.

"Yes, he does seem in trouble," said the child's companion, an elderly gentleman, evidently a clergyman.

"Shall we ride across and ask him what is the matter?"

"Oh, yes! do let us," was the ready answer.

In a few seconds the two had ascended the hill-side and were within hail of the shepherd, who, worn out by the exertions he had made, had sunk down on the soft green grass, grumbling aloud, "It is of no use, they must take their own way!"

"Well, Roger, what's wrong with you?" shouted the clergyman.

The old man lifted himself up, and seeing who it was addressing him, rose, touched his cap, and went over to where the riders had stopped their horses.

"Please, your reverence," he said, "there's no doing anything with them sheep, they be just so skittish, the old as well as the young, I'm a-thinking it's the spring, just look at 'em!" And with a deprecating gesture he glanced at his flock—the young lambs gambolling far and wide on the green hill-side, followed by their mothers, whose loud "baa-as" had no more effect in retaining these very disobedient little ones, than the shepherd's voice had had.

"But where's Cap?" asked the little girl.

"Ah! that's just all the mischief, Missey. Cap's done for! And them cunning things they knows it."

"Cap done for! Do you mean to say he's dead?" exclaimed the clergyman.

"It be pretty much as if he were," answered the old

man, sadly. "I'd rather he were, then I shouldn't have to do it!"

"Do what, Roger?" asked the child.

"Why, hang him, Missey, that's about all," he answered doggedly.

"Hang Cap? your dear, good Cap—there's not a better sheep-dog on the downs, Roger!" exclaimed the Vicar.

"I know it, sir, but he 'aint of no more use to me, and we poor folks can't keep useless mouths to feed; I must get another dog, Cap can't work no more."

"Why, a week ago I saw him running after the sheep as actively as possible; what has happened since?"

"Some boys got to throwing stones, and one hit Cap on the leg and smashed it up; he just crawled into the hut, and there he have lain ever since a-moaning, not able to move, till it makes my heart ache. It would be a kindness to put him out of his pain, and I've made up my mind to do it to-night."

"Oh, Roger, how can you! He may get well still," exclaimed the little girl, her eyes full of tears.

"If he'd been for getting better, he'd have shown signs of mending before now, Miss Florence; and he's worser, why, his leg were as big well nigh as my head this morning when I left him, and he don't eat, only drink, he's never done drinking."

"Probably he knows what's best for him," answered the Vicar. "Animals are often wiser than men, their instincts tell them what is good for them. Anyway, I am sorry for your trouble, Roger; Cap was a good dog, and I'm afraid you'll have some trouble in replacing him."

"I'm afraid so too, your reverence, thank you

kindly!" and the old shepherd pulled his forelock. "Good-day, Missey," he continued, "and don't you be for vexing yourself; you see we must all die, and dogs aint no exception," and he patted the neck of the pony.

"Good-bye, Roger, I'm very sorry," was the gentle answer, and her brown eyes looked very sad as she nodded her head in token of farewell and followed her companion down the hillside to regain the high road.

The shepherd watched her for a minute or two, then, as he turned back to his scattered flock, he muttered, "She have a good heart, have Miss Florence, let it be for man or beast."

The little girl and the Vicar rode on for some time in silence; at last the latter said:—

"I wonder whether the dog is as bad as Roger thinks, Florence? These country people know so little about doctoring themselves, much less their animals. A stone may have injured the leg, but hardly to the extent of smashing it up as he seems to say."

"Let's go and see!" said Florence, eagerly. "Roger's cottage is only out yonder," and she pointed to a group of cottages nestling under the hillside.

"We may as well," answered the Vicar. "The dog was a valuable animal, and very intelligent. I often noticed him. It would be a pity to kill him if there were any chance of his recovery."

Once more they turned their horses' heads, and rode up the lane leading to the cottages.

Florence sprang lightly off her pony, tried the latch of the last cottage in the row, but to her dismay the door was locked; from within came a low, angry bark, followed by a moan of pain.

"Roger's locked him in!" she said, returning disconsolately to where her companion, not yet dismounted, was waiting for her.

"I'm sorry for that," said the Vicar. "Of course, he's taken the key with him. Well, Florence, I'm afraid we must leave poor Cap to his fate!"

At that moment the next cottage door opened, and a woman with a baby in her arms, and a small boy of about seven half hiding behind her, stepped out. She curtseyed, saying:—

"Roger be out, your reverence, he's after his sheep, and a precious sight of trouble he'll have with them. Cap's a-dying!"

"He makes noise enough still," said the Vicar, as the dog continued to bark at intervals. "It's to see Cap we've come, Mrs. Norton, but the door is locked, so our visit is useless. How's your husband?"

"Better, sir, thank you; he came out of the Infirmary last week, and is picking up nicely; but if it's Cap you want to see, your reverence, my Jimmy knows where the key is hid, and he'll take you into the place. Cap won't let no stranger go in, not though he be dying; but he knows Jimmy, who gives him to drink. The poor beast is so mighty thirsty."

"That's well, come Jimmy, my lad, find the key and let us in," said the Vicar.

The little chap, who needed no second bidding, brought the key forth, put it into the lock, and opening the door, called out, softly, "Cap, Cap, it's all right, friends." The dog growled, and tried to lift himself up, as the Vicar and Florence entered. The little girl went fearlessly up to where he lay, saying, in a soft, caressing tone, "Poor Cap, poor Cap!" It was enough, he looked up with his speaking brown eyes, now bloodshot and full of pain, into her face; and did not resent it when, kneeling down beside him, she stroked, with her little ungloved hand, the large, intelligent head.

To the Vicar he was rather less amenable, but by dint of coaxing he at last allowed him to touch and examine the wounded leg, Jimmy and Florence persuasively telling him it was "all right." Indeed the latter was on the floor beside him, with his head on her lap, keeping up a continuous murmur, much as a mother does over a sick child.

"Well," said the Vicar, rising from his examination, "as far as I can tell there are no broken bones; the leg is badly bruised, it ought to be fomented, to take the inflammation and swelling down."

"How do you foment?" asked Florence.

"With hot cloths dipped into boiling water," answered the Vicar.

"Then that's quite easy. I'll stay here and do it. Now, Jimmy, let's get sticks and make the kettle boil."

There was no hesitation in the child's manner—she was told what ought to be done and she set about doing it as a simple matter of course.

"But they will be expecting you at home," said the Vicar.

"Not if you tell them I am here," answered Florence; "and my sister and one of the maids can come and fetch me home in time for tea, and," she hesitated, "they had better bring some old flannel and cloths, there does not seem to be much here; but you will wait and show me how to foment, won't you?"

"Well, yes," said the Vicar, carried away by the quick energy of the little girl.

EARLY DAYS. 17

And soon the fire was lit and the water boiling; an old smock frock of the shepherd's had been discovered in a corner, which Florence had deliberately torn in

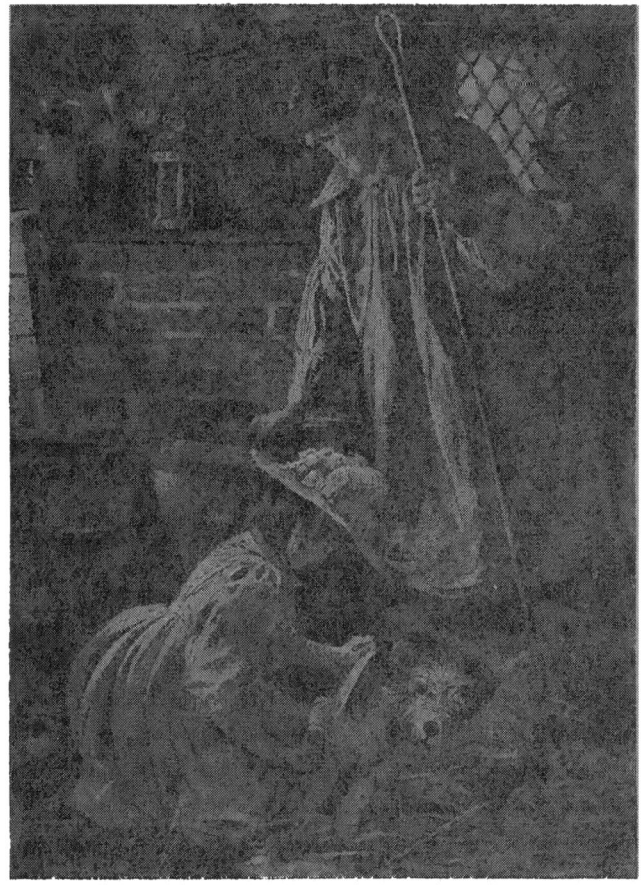

FLORENCE NIGHTINGALE'S FIRST "CASE."

pieces, and to the Vicar's remark, "What will Roger say?" she answered, "We'll give him another." And so Florence Nightingale made her first compress and spent the whole of that bright spring day in nursing her first patient—the shepherd's dog.

In the evening when Roger came, not expecting to find visitors in his humble cottage, and dangling a bit of cord in his hand, Florence went up to him. "You can throw that away, Roger," she said, "your dog won't die, look at him!" and Cap rose and crawled towards his master, whining with pleasure.

"Deary me! deary me! What have you done to him, Miss Florence? He could not move this morning when I left him."

Then Florence told Roger, and explained the mode of treatment. "You have only to go on just to-night, and to-morrow he will be almost well, the Vicar says." And smiling brightly, she continued, "Mrs. Norton has promised to see to Cap to-morrow, when you are out, so now you need not kill him, he will soon be able to do his work again."

"Thank you kindly, Missey, I do indeed," said the old man, huskily. "It went hard with me to do away with him; but what can a poor man do?" and putting out his hand he stroked the dog.

"I'll see to him, Missey, now as I knows what is to be done," and he stood his crook in the corner and hung his cap up on the peg.

Then Florence took her leave, stroking and petting the dog to the last, and those who, standing at the cottage door, watched her disappear, little thought they were gazing upon one whose mission would be to tend the sick and wounded in the great battle-field of life, and how, in years to come, men dying far away from home would raise themselves upon their pillows to "kiss her shadow as it passed by."

* * * * *

EARLY DAYS.

On the 13th of May, 1820, Florence Nightingale was born, and named Florence, after that lovely city on the banks of the Arno, which was her birthplace. It is a day worthy of note, especially for women, for it marks an epoch in their development, and in their position, as regards the world, and their individual work in the world. She was the younger of Mr. William Shore Nightingale's two daughters. Her father was a wealthy landowner, squire of "Embley Park," Hampshire, and "Lea Hurst," Derbyshire.

The Shores of Derbyshire are of very ancient descent. Lord Teignmouth is the representative of another branch of the same family.

Mr. William Shore assumed his mother's name of Nightingale in the year 1819, at which date he inherited her fortune.

The Manor of " Lea Hurst," where the greater part of the early youth and womanhood of Florence Nightingale was passed, was held as far back as the reign of King John by the Alveleys, who, in the early part of the 13th century erected there a chapel. It is very beautifully situated, in the centre of the Matlock district, about two miles from Cromford station.

If, as it is very commonly stated, our characters, and to a certain extent our after-lives, are influenced by our early surroundings and associations, then, truly, Florence Nightingale was highly favoured.

Born in the " city of flowers," her love of flowers amounted almost to a passion. She considered their influence as most beneficial in the sick chamber, and it is owing to this strong predilection on her part that the hospital wards no longer wear the dreary forlorn aspect so uniform in days gone by, but are made gay with flowers ; and that year after year in our churches " Hospital Sunday " is a day of joy and brightness, when Christ's little ones come laden with Earth's fairest flowers for His sick, and His "heavy laden."

It seems almost as if every variety of landscape must have surrounded the home of our heroine. In the distance wonderful views of the Peak country, grey gritstone rocks ; and near at hand the river Derwent running through green pastures, close by the stately Elizabethan Hall built in the form of a cross, and embosomed in a profusion of beautiful trees. Lea Hurst is no ordinary dwelling-house ; it stands forth, visible from afar, on the sloping hillside! The stately gateway, with massive posts on either side, terminated with globes of stone, has an air of mediæval grandeur. It is built, as we have said before, in the form of a cross, with gables at its extremities and its sides ; surmounted with hip knobs and ball terminations. The windows, which open beneath the many gables, are square, headed with drip stones and stone mullions. Very effective is the cluster of strongly built chimney stacks which rise from the roof, they convey to the mind an impression of warmth and hospitality.

The garden lies at the back, as also a long avenue of trees, a favourite resort of Florence Nightingale in her childhood, because there she found amusement and companionship combined. A great number of squirrels made the trees in the avenue their home, leaping from branch to branch, looking down upon the passers-by with their keen brown eyes. To them the little maiden was a familiar friend, they knew her well, and

"LEA HURST," WHERE FLORENCE NIGHTINGALE SPENT HER EARLY YEARS.

would come tumbling down almost at her feet, when she made her appearance with her pockets full of nuts, which she let fall amongst them, laughing at their eagerness, their little quarrels, and their funny ways. They felt no fear of her, but greeted her coming with the little familiar cry peculiar to them.

Wherever Florence went the same glad welcome awaited her. Hers was a familiar presence in the poor cottages around her home, especially when there was sickness or trouble therein; sometimes in the company of the vicar of the parish, who had studied medicine, and from whom her first notions of hygiene were derived; sometimes as her mother's almoner, taking food and clothes to those who stood in need; but what they valued perhaps more even than the material gifts she brought was the gentle presence, the delicate touch of the child's hand on the aching head, the serious face so full of sympathy, and the soft voice speaking words of encouragement and hope. "A Ministering Angel," even while she still stood on the threshold of life, her child's soul was touched by the pains and sorrows of those around her.

Not of common mould was Florence Nightingale, her mission was born with her. It came naturally to her to bear other's burdens, to lighten the weight of sin and sorrow, the knowledge of which grew with her growth, screened and sheltered though she was by the love of many in her beautiful home.

But love "makes abler to love," and in this atmosphere her heart and soul developed, not suddenly, but gradually, like all things else in nature— the bud, the blossom, and at last the full blown flower.

Mr. William Shore Nightingale was himself a highly cultivated man and a great traveller. It was but natural, therefore, that he should desire his daughters to receive a thoroughly careful education, and he provided for this by every means in his power.

The next few years, passed by Florence Nightingale and her sister in the schoolroom, and occasionally in foreign travel, were uneventful. We all know the quiet routine a well-conducted education entails. The two sisters studied seriously, and grew up well-informed, accomplished women, good musicians, and in every respect fitted to adorn the position in the world to which their birth and wealth entitled them.

But society, by which I mean purely worldly society, could have little or no charms for such a nature as our heroine's. Its shallowness must have come home to her at a very early stage. Her own standard of right was so elevated that she must necessarily have experienced a feeling akin to pain, when she came into contact with every-day humanity.

Moreover, there was in her character a natural love of work—a desire to be up and doing for the good of others. Living from her earliest childhood amongst the poor, she realised, almost before she was aware of the fact, how great their ignorance was in all domestic matters, and their utter helplessness in times of sickness. The intense desire she felt of assisting them made this ignorance even more apparent to her, and enabled her to see more clearly the evil effects of it.

To remedy this evil was her next thought; and how to a great extent she succeeded in so doing, her whole life story, from girlhood to womanhood, and to the end of her life, bears testimony.

CHAPTER II.

"AN EXAMPLE."

> "Let our increasing earnest prayer,
> Be, too, for light—for strength to bear
> Our portion of the weight of care,
> That crushes into dumb despair
> One half the human race."—*Longfellow*.

WHAT was the cause of disease and suffering, and how could they be alleviated? Such were the questions which now unceasingly occupied Florence Nightingale's mind and heart, and to the solution of which she at last resolved to devote her whole life. Her family, whilst it did not actually oppose her inclinations, gave her little encouragement, but her vocation was marked, and they could not fail to recognise it. Several members of her family being attacked by long and dangerous illnesses, it came naturally to her to constitute herself their nurse. She just showed herself in society, and then disappeared. Her whole soul was set upon higher, more ennobling work, and how to prepare herself for it grew to be the object of her daily life.

When we are possessed by one absorbing thought or feeling, it is difficult to create in ourselves an interest for, or participate in, pleasures which have a wholly different tendency. The effort is a weariness to the spirit—it was even so with Florence Nightingale; in the midst of the gaieties of the world she remembered her poorer brethren, the sick and the untended, and she yearned after them. In the brilliant saloon she thought of the dark and dreary attics where the uncared for of the earth lay dying; and day by day, almost hour by hour, the powerful impetus of, we may truly call it, a Divine calling drove her forth into the path she was destined to tread.

Naturally, what lay nearest home, first met with her attention; she spent much of her time in visiting the hospitals in her own county, studying their organisation, and making herself acquainted, as far as was possible, with their discipline and working powers. From thence she proceeded to London, and pursued the same mode of careful investigation and study. It was at this critical period of her life that she made the acquaintance of Mrs. Elizabeth Fry, whose career of philanthropy was fast drawing to a close.

She had laboured long and earnestly in a field still more arid than the one which attracted Florence Nightingale, and her work had not been without its reward even in this world. Truly the aged woman, whose rest was so near at hand, must have felt herself strangely drawn towards her young sister, just starting upon her arduous labours; there was a bond of union between them almost stronger than the ties of blood—that love for suffering humanity of which Christ set the first and great example.

> "The air is full of farewells to the dying,
> And moanings for the dead."

But what of the living? From hospitals and prison-houses the cry for help ascended, too often, alas, in vain, unheard in the rush and turmoil of the world, because none were listening.

A few only heard the wailing and responded to the call—Elizabeth Fry, John Howard, Florence Nightingale. It came to them as if it had been Christ's own voice bidding them arise and tend His forsaken ones; and, hearing, they obeyed and went forth in His name to do what they could. A blessed band! A holy calling—to dispel darkness, to raise the lost, and to bring the light of God where ignorance, sin, and misery reigned supreme!

Miss Nightingale was from the first aware that before she could teach others she must herself understand the work she wished them to accomplish; she felt the absolute necessity of acquiring for herself a practical knowledge of sickness and disease in their various forms, and the right and, therefore, the most efficacious way of tending the sick. Gradually she devoted her whole time to this study.

After spending some months in the London hospitals, she visited similar establishments in Dublin and Edinburgh, examining into the minutest details of hospital life. Then she went abroad to France, Germany, and Italy, and pursued the same systematic investigations. She was not long in perceiving wherein lay the great mistake in English hospital organisation, and in the nursing of our sick. On the Continent from time immemorial there had existed societies, the members of which were entirely devoted to the service of the hospitals, or to tending the sick in their own houses. They were not paid, it was their life, their religion. They were the servants of God, and as such bound to serve His creatures. Of this class in France and Italy are the Sisters of St. Vincent de Paul, who, in their grey uniforms and white coifs, are the recognised nurses of the poor, and the helpers of all who need help. In Protestant Germany there are the Deaconesses, more especially the institution created by Pastor Fliedner at Kaiserwerth, where nurses were especially trained and sent forth far and wide to do their work amongst the sick, and to raise the fallen.

This establishment exercised such a marked influence upon Florence Nightingale—the spirit of the founder was so entirely in accordance with her own, that it will, I think, be hardly out of place here to give our readers a slight sketch of the life of Pastor Fliedner, and the truly wonderful work which he accomplished. He was one of the pioneers of social reform of the nineteenth century, and, as we shall see, served as guide and mentor to her who was destined to a high calling in the world of philanthropy.

Theodore Fliedner was born in January, 1800, at Eppstein, a small village on the frontiers of Hesse and Nassau, where his father was a parish clergyman. He was not a brilliant scholar, and never throughout his career did he make any mark by his theological attainments, though Germany was then, as it is now, a vast field of controversy; from all of which Theodore Fliedner kept aloof. His work lay in an entirely different groove. At the age of twenty he passed his final examination, and became Pastor of the Evangelical Church at Kaiserwerth, a little town on the Rhine, some few miles from Dusseldorf. Nothing could be

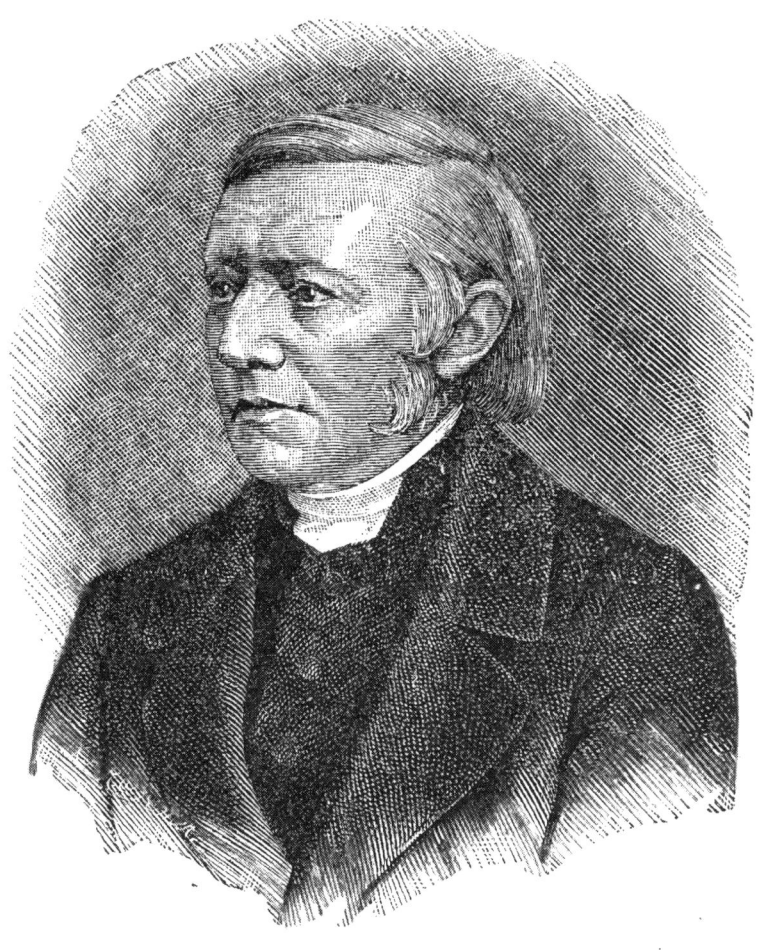

less inviting than the aspect of this town—dirt, solitude and poverty being its chief characteristics; the Rhine indeed flows past it broad and rapid, but neither boat nor landing-place were there to make it available. It was in this obscure corner of the world that the young pastor began his ministration, receiving for all remuneration the stipend of £27 per annum.

Goldsmith tells us of the parish priest

"Passing rich with forty pounds a year,"

and though we may take into consideration that life in Germany was then, as it is now, cheaper and simpler than in England, still so small an income could barely have sufficed, with the strictest economy and self-denial, for the necessaries of life. The population, almost wholly Roman Catholic, was very wretched, very dirty, and very diseased. It seems marvellous that out of such materials the energy of one Christian mind should succeed in raising so vast and noble an institution as the one we are attempting to describe. The apparent hopelessness of the situation may perhaps have served to stimulate the young man's energies. Come what might, matters could not be worse than they were, anything was better than the state of stagnation and misery in which he found his flock. He had been amongst them but a short time when his small income was further diminished by the failure of the velvet manufactures, which supplied a large proportion of the members of his congregation with work, and the young pastor cast about in his mind how he should provide for the endowment of his church and the necessities of his poorer neighbours. He undertook journeys for this purpose through Germany, Holland, and England, pleaded his own cause, and met with considerable success. Probably it was at this time that the name of John Howard reached his ears, for he turned his attention to prison reform in Germany, where the prisons were, if possible, in a worse state than in England, the wretched inmates being huddled together in dirty rooms, badly fed, and left in complete idleness. He went so far as to ask to be imprisoned himself for some time, in order that he might judge prison life from experience. This request, however, was refused, but he was allowed to hold fortnightly services in the Dusseldorf prison, and to visit the inmates individually. Thus the first stone was laid, and a band of men, imbued with the same interest, gradually cemented their union, and on the 18th of June, 1826, the first Prison Society in Germany was founded. But once the men and women, upon whom prison life had left its mark, were again let loose upon the world, with the mark of Cain so to speak upon their brows, whither were they to go? what was to become of them? This great social question presented itself to Pastor Fliedner's mind in all its vastness; he had no money and no means; he could not well expose his young wife and children to hourly contact with sin and shame, and yet if he could but rescue one lost sheep from perdition! Was he not the shepherd of Christ's sheep? How should he answer his Master when He claimed them at his hand if they were lost? In the garden which surrounded his own humble home was a summer house, and here he set to work, labouring with his own hands, planning and devising, until he had made it a shelter from rain and wind, habitable in fact; in it he placed a bed, a table, and a chair, and one day he brought thither a woman, a Magdalene, just lately released from prison, and who, as she stepped beyond its gates and stood once more face to face with the cruel world, had shivered, and turning her dim eyes, so long unaccustomed to the free light of day, towards him had murmured, "Where shall I go?" Ah, where indeed! who in the wide world would have the moral courage to hold out the hand of fellowship to the fallen? It was so easy to bid her "go and sin no more," but the ways and means? when every door is closed, and every face turned another way!

"If you will follow me, I will take you home." Was it a man or an angel speaking to her? She questioned not but followed him, in simple faith, to the poor home he had prepared for her, and there she found rest and peace for her wounded soul, weary of sin and unrest. And the story spread abroad; it took place in the year 1833, and others came seeking the same shelter, the same protection, and thus the Penitentiary grew; the seed cast into the ground took root and flourished, and became a mighty tree, spreading forth its branches far and wide, to shelter those who truly longed to "sin no more." From henceforth there was a home at Kaiserwerth for discharged female convicts, money came in, a separate building was devoted to the purpose, standing in its own garden and fields, capable of receiving from fifteen to twenty females, but, and here we see the comprehensive charity and delicacy of the founder, it was, and is still, the only part of the establishment not open to the inspection of strangers.

Imbued with Divine love, Pastor Fliedner understood the sacredness of true sorrow and true repentance, and suffered not strangers to gaze thereon with idle curiosity.

In the same year, 1833, in a deserted manufactory, the establishment of which, with its Protestant workmen, was the first cause of Mr. Fliedner's presence at Kaiserwerth, the hospital was begun, also with one patient. It contains now over one hundred beds. But a hospital without nurses was an anomaly which presented itself clearly to the common sense of the founder, and he recognised the fact that if his work was to succeed it needed female influence to be brought to bear upon it. In this nineteenth century the social influence of woman has made itself most particularly felt. Queens and Queen Regents are reigning over the lords of the creation from Tahiti to the British Isles; never before was the co-operative union of the two sexes so mutually influential upon the march of society. Only in our greatest need of all, religious need, has this co-operation been the least courted. Woman had so far been left to isolated efforts, tending at once to show her extreme fitness, her impotence without the guiding hand of man, and, also, the power of union. The great defect in the system of the "Sœurs de Charité" in the Romish Church is their extreme docility, which yields them up as mere instruments under the system and administration to which they belong. Whatever fault is to be found with them arises from their teachers, not from themselves. Their influence is immense, but Kaiserwerth has shown the world how, under a different system, the faults might be avoided, and the influence gained.

It was with all this in his mind, and feeling the

"AN EXAMPLE."

absolute necessity of woman's tact and subtle influence, that he founded the order of deaconesses, or rather, as the name implies, he revived, in this strictly Protestant Institution, an order which the Primitive Church recognised as necessary for the proper working of her system. Candidates for the office of deaconess received the Church's solemn blessing before they entered upon their work. They were henceforth to consider themselves the servants of the Lord Jesus, the servants of the sick and poor, and the servants of each other. They were fettered by no vows. Their engagement was for five years, but a deaconess was free to leave at any moment. They were solemnly consecrated by the imposition of hands, and the pastor's final blessing pronounced in these words :—

"May God the Father, the Son, and the Holy Ghost, Three Persons in one God, bless you; may He stablish you in the Truth until death, and give you hereafter the Crown of Life. Amen."

Thus though bound they were free; if a deaconess found herself unequal to the task she had undertaken, if she were called upon to return to her parents or relations; or even might she be disposed to marry—for a deaconess is not supposed to have unfitted herself for the duties of wife or mother—she could go; only Mr. Fliedner considered that her new duties were in that case incompatible with her continuing a deaconess. A French protestant pastor, differing from him on this point, Mr. Fliedner smiled as he put the practical objection: "If I, her spiritual director and head, ordered her to go where duty might call her, and her temporal lord and master commanded her to stay, whom should she obey?" No deaconess was to be under twenty-five years of age. The dress was simple but not unbecoming, a blue cotton gown, white apron, collar and muslin cap, without any peculiarity of shape; it has the great advantage, that out of doors it attracts no particular attention to the wearer. One thing is certain, from this time forward Mr. Fliedner's work prospered, as he himself in his most sanguine mood had never deemed possible; his whole heart and soul were absorbed in his work. Everything was done decently, in order, and with knowledge. The deaconesses were trained for nursing and for teaching, for between the years 1836 and 1847, there were added to the original establishment an infant school, a normal school for training infant school mistresses, an orphanage for girls of the middle class, and an asylum for female lunatics.

But it must be borne in mind that all these institutions were subordinate to the one great object which the pastor never lost sight of, namely, the forming of deaconesses; this he felt was the pivot upon which the whole work depended, to supply young females of a religious tone of mind with such mental discipline and practical knowledge as should make them far more useful servants of Christ than they could be without it. Of course the far greater number are employed in their own country and amongst their own people; but to a true philanthropist all men are his brethren, and Pastor Fliedner was in this no exception; moreover, he was perhaps desirous like Lycurgus of testing the stability of his work when his guiding hand should be removed from the helm, therefore, as soon as he judged that these numerous institutions had taken root at Kaiserwerth and were in full working order, he determined to withdraw, for a time at least, his presence from amongst them, and

KAISERWERTH.

leave it in higher hands than his either to stand or fall.

In 1849 he resigned his pastoral charge at Kaiserwerth, and set forth for the purpose of founding "mother houses" all over the world. At Constantinople, London, and the United States he opened establishments, as also at Smyrna, Alexandria, and Bucharest. In April, 1851, the pastor himself accompanied four deaconesses to Jerusalem, and there founded a branch establishment on Mount Sion, to nurse the sick of all creeds, and form a school for Christian instructresses and nurses in the East. The king of Prussia made them a gift of a house, which now contains a hospital, seminary, and hospice. "Many sick," writes one of the sisters, "are now under our care. We have always many applications from without; persons with sore fingers, feet and eyes, come, just as if a wonder-working doctor lived here; I wash their hands and feet with soap and water, etc., etc." The sisters exercise an influence over the female Orientals in particular, which can never be obtained by male instructors. Little Oriental children are consigned to their care—at one time they had two Arabian girls from Hebron and one from Tafet. And so it grew and prospered.

But for him who had laboured so long and so earnestly in his Master's vineyard the end was gradually approaching. He returned to Europe, and never flagged in the work which had become a necessity to him; but his active life was over, and doubtless the sense of physical weakness which was creeping over him made him long for rest. And he remembered the many who had fought the "good fight" and like himself were weary with the battle of life—for them also he provided, it was his last creation, "The House of Evening Rest," for retired deaconesses at Kaiserwerth. There, where his labour of love had begun, from whence they whom he had trained had gone forth in simple faith like the disciples of old to preach the Gospel by precept and example, he bade them come home again, when their strength failed them and their eyes grew dim, to rest beneath the shadow of the flag of the institution, which on *fête* days floated from an adjoining tower and on which was pictured "a dove bearing an olive branch," and the same emblem of peace which rested on Noah's ark as it tossed on the troubled waters is sculptured over the entrance to the little chapel, which has indeed proved an ark of refuge to many weary souls tossed to and fro upon the waves of this "troublesome world."

When this, his last active work was accomplished his rest was very near; the shadows of death, through which he was to enter into the New Jerusalem, were gathering around him. The human frame was worn out caring for others, but the imperishable intellect and spirit were clear and strong to the very end. When at last unable to leave his room he still continued to carry on a voluminous correspondence. On the 4th of October, 1864, he gently breathed his last, leaving behind him to testify to his work 100 stations attended by 430 deaconesses!

CHAPTER III.

IN TRAINING.

"Go and do thou likewise."

IT was in the steps of that admirable man, Pastor Fliedner, that Florence Nightingale determined to follow. In England we had as yet no such institution as he had founded, and there seemed no likelihood of any improvement in the accepted system of nursing. The need might be, and doubtless was felt, but it required considerable energy to break through old accepted routine and organise a new order of things. Above all, union was necessary, isolated cases of neglect and even death arising from bad nursing were not sufficient to arouse a whole nation to demand a radical reform. Custom and habit are, as is well known, difficult to break through.

It is true that a sick-nurse was at this time held in the very lowest estimation, and she was generally of a stamp which authorized the feelings of dislike, we might almost say of fear, which she inspired. The "Sairey Gamp" type was not likely to inspire confidence. These women were generally of a low class, and unfit by reason of age or infirmity to earn their living in any active, honourable manner, being for the most part addicted to that worst of all vices —drink. To leave our dear ones in such hands, surely it is to aggravate the pangs of sickness and of death! and yet it is a fact that outside their own circle, in cases of emergency, the rich could command nothing better, money was powerless where ignorance reigned supreme. What then must have been the fate of the poor?

With this deplorable state of things ever before her, Florence Nightingale went from city to city, throughout Europe, seeking a remedy, not allowing herself to be prejudiced by caste, religion, or race. As Pastor Fliedner wandered among the prisoners and captives, among the sick and the weary, even so did she.

The hospitals of Berlin, and many others in Germany, those of Paris, Lyons, Rome, Alexandria, Constantinople, and Brussels were visited by her. She examined every different system, and compared one with the other. In a valuable book which she wrote many years later, in 1863, entitled "Notes on Hospitals," she has given all this vast experience to the world. She especially dwells upon the construction of hospitals, a point to which little importance was attached in earlier times. The block system evidently meets with her highest approbation. She writes almost enthusiastically of the way this is conceived and carried out in the famous Laboisière Hospital in Paris, and mentions as a curious fact that though this was, at the time she wrote, one of the best hospitals in the world, it was yielding one of the highest rates of mortality, owing to its being heated and ventilated by artificial means. So much for personal and theoretical knowledge, but Florence Nightingale knew that more than this was needed—that she must be able practically to carry out what she had seen and heard, if she were ever really to be called upon to do so.

It was a great step to take—one involving much self-sacrifice, and which her naturally delicate health rendered even more difficult; but nevertheless she did not shrink from her self-imposed task, or from the self-sacrifice which the carrying out of it entailed.

At two different periods of her life she took up her residence at Kaiserwerth, and remained there for several months. At once she recognised that she had found what she had so long sought — a spirit of devotion, of order, and unity of purpose. It was impossible not to be impressed with the air of purity and deep, unaffected piety which pervaded the whole place; and yet there was no asceticism, it was the world, and yet not the world in the ordinary sense of the word. There was the mother, Madame Fliedner, the pastor's wife, mother of his large family, laying no claim to the dignity of "Lady Superior," but a plain Christian woman who had not found the duties of wife and mother incompatible with spiritual cares, when both alike were exercised under one and the same guide and director, her husband. There were the young deaconesses with their intelligent, animated countenances, no mere instruments yielding a blind and passive obedience, but voluntary and enlightened agents, obeying, on conviction, an inward principle

In 1849 she enrolled herself as voluntary nurse in this establishment, and thus became practically acquainted with every form of disease and of the whole system of nursing. From henceforth she understood her work in its very minutest details.

To fully appreciate the strength of mind and the determination necessary for a young and accomplished woman like Miss Nightingale to pursue such a career, it must be remembered that it was a path yet untrodden, one for which, in England at least, little or no sympathy was felt ; that to attain her end Florence Nightingale had, therefore, to break through prejudices both social and religious. It was impossible that the generality of people should understand the motives which made her, a young and highly gifted woman, in the full enjoyment of all the good things of this world, deliberately turn away from the pleasures of society, which she was so well fitted to adorn, and voluntarily devote herself to the "weary and the heavy laden," taking up their burdens as if they had been her own. Florence Nightingale may truly be ranked amongst the reformers of the nineteenth century, and like all reformers she had to bear with misinterpretation, with the sneer of ignorance, and the impossibility of making narrow intellects and small minds understand and accept new ideas, new modes of action, at a moment's notice. That a lady could move out of her own immediate circle, that she was destined for anything more serious in life than to grace a drawing-room, was an innovation new to many. The principle of the nobility of woman's work was in its infancy, and a certain slur rested upon those who either from necessity or from any personal motive enrolled themselves among the workers. Miss Nightingale chose to ignore this feeling and went her way quietly and earnestly, as

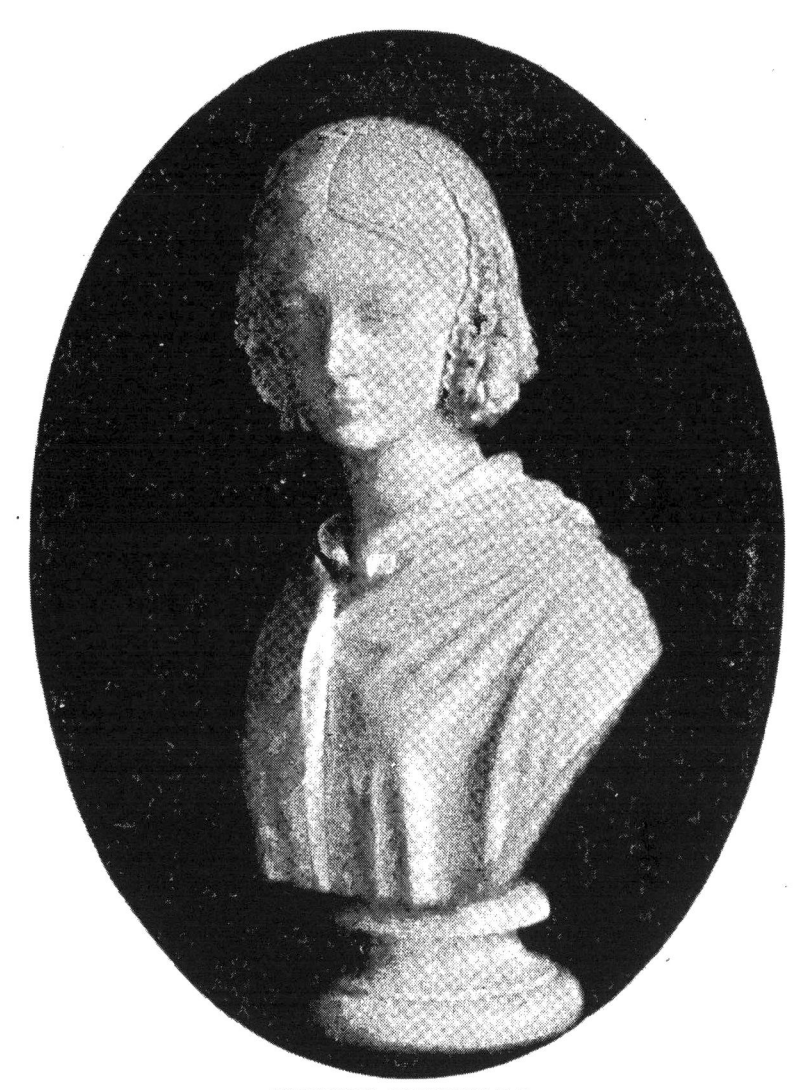

FLORENCE NIGHTINGALE.

From a white marble Bust by Sir John Steel, a personal friend of Miss Nightingale, and paid for by Penny Subscriptions by the Soldiers engaged in the Crimean War.

IN TRAINING.   47

one who has an object to attain—an object in her own estimation so high, so noble, that no counter opinion could affect her.

Her personal appearance was in keeping with her character. Her eyes were especially brilliant and penetrating, her general demeanour quiet and reserved. She was essentially a graceful woman, upon whom it was impossible to look without applying to her the words of the poet:—

> "A being breathing thoughtful breath,
> A traveller betwixt life and death ;
> The reason firm, the temperate will,
> Endurance, foresight, strength, and skill ;
> A perfect woman, nobly planned,
> To warn, to comfort, and command ;
> And yet a spirit, still and bright,
> With something of an angel light."

Her power of self-restraint was, even in these early days of initiative work, remarkable, as also the nerve she invariably displayed when attending the sick. Some people imagine that it is want of feeling, a defect in the moral organisation of a woman, when she can quietly stand by, witness and assist at an operation ; it is, on the contrary, a gift not given to all, and of great value. Looking back on the Franco-Prussian war, the writer of these pages can but remember how woman's help was sought for and esteemed in public and private ambulances, and for all ordinary hospital work. In that terrible winter of 1870, when whole provinces of France were little more than great battlefields, when the wounded and the dying came crawling into the towns or lay huddled together at the railway stations, just- as the poor, too often maimed, creatures had been taken out of the trucks and laid down upon the bare floor; then it was that women's help was sought, and they came gladly to the fore, to do what they could. Ignorant only too often, but tender and pitiful. How gladly they were welcomed by both doctors and soldiers, and how, in that great emergency, weak hands grew strong for very pity's sake, only those who were present and lived through those awful days can tell.

We live from day to day ignorant of what the morrow may bring forth, therefore it is that no lesson or experience should be allowed to escape our observation; we cannot tell when the need for using it may come to us.

Most assuredly Florence Nightingale could have had no foreshadowing of the future, or of the task which lay before her, and yet she neglected nothing to perfect herself in the line of life she had mapped out for herself. Europe was at peace, as it had seldom been before; for forty years England's sword was sheathed, and there was nothing to lead one to suppose that her soldiers would be called upon to draw it forth; and even if war broke out she could not for one moment surmise that she of all others, a weak woman, would be called upon to play a conspicuous part in it —yet such was the case, a great war was looming over Europe, and she, unknowingly, was preparing herself for her post. In every action of her life Miss Nightingale followed a natural instinct, born in her, part of her own being, and which had grown and developed with her growth. Having served, as we have shown, at Kaiserwerth until she had acquired full knowledge and experience of her work, she next went to Paris and took up her residence with the Sisters of St. Vincent de Paul. The work of this community lies entirely in the hospitals, orphanages, and foundling hospitals. The experience she gained whilst thus employed must have been very great; unfortunately she fell seriously ill, but she was thus enabled to speak warmly and from experience of the intelligent care with which the sisters nursed her back to health. One thing above all others presented itself as a tangible fact to her, the keynote to the whole system.

The Sisters of St. Vincent de Paul, like the Deaconesses of Kaiserwerth, were women set apart, whose whole lives belonged to others, who did not look upon the nursing of their sick brethren as a pecuniary speculation, but as a work to be done for Christ's sake in the spirit of love and self-sacrifice. Large minded, as all truly religious men and women must needs be, she recognised that difference of doctrine could in no wise influence the spirit which animated this class of labourers in Christ's vineyard. Love was their motive power, in self-abnegation lay their strength. They did not cut themselves off from the world, on the contrary they lived in it, and for it. In the crowded alleys, in the hospital wards, and wherever there was sin, sorrow, or suffering, there these women were to be found, treading softly, with knowledge and experience at their command, and with no objects, no aims, outside their round of daily work. Their homes were with their patients, they were not here to-day and gone to-morrow, as the whim of the moments or the love of money might dictate.

And sadly Florence Nightingale acknowledged that in this respect England was behind her neighbours; we had no such institutions, and at the time there seemed no opening for such work—fathers, and brothers, and mothers, would have risen up in arms at the very idea of their daughters and sisters being trained for sick-nurses. It would have been viewed, as when it really came to pass it was viewed, as indelicate for gently nurtured women to witness and assist at the loathsome sights of the operating room or hospital wards. It needed a hard lesson to bring English men and women to acknowledge that wherever there is suffering there must needs be work, that the claims of humanity break down all barriers, that neither birth nor education can or ought to exempt women from this field of labour; on the contrary, wealth and education are prerogatives, and ought to render their possessors the more fitting to help those who are less favoured. Intellect and refinement are never so powerful as when brought to bear upon the ignorant or suffering, the most menial services wear a different aspect when gentleness and loving kindness, not mercenary motives, guide both hand and eye.

There is no doubt that Florence Nightingale had long been aware of all this from her own experience, but perhaps the greatest wisdom of all, and the most difficult to put into practice, is to wait, and this she was able to do, because, modest and retiring in no ordinary degree, it would have been against her principles to attempt to impose her opinions on the world at large, by preaching an open crusade against the errors of the times. She contented herself by working out her theories privately, for the benefit of her own immediate circle. She had no desire for self glorification, her own personality was merged in her desire to help and succour those who could not help themselves; and this is most certainly the secret of both hers and Pastor Fliedner's success in their undertakings; they had no second thought, no—as the French express it so graphically—"*Arrière pensée.*" Their knowledge of the needs of the human race absorbed their every thought, and they were possessed of one desire—the amelioration of those evils which they both saw and felt acutely, and to remedy which they were ready to sacrifice their whole lives.

Upon her return from Paris, Miss Nightingale spent some months in her own beautiful home, surrounded by friends and relations, who rejoiced in her society, and would gladly have detained her amongst them. But the spirit of Christ's words, though unexpressed, was ever present with her, "Wist ye not that I must be about my Father's business?" After, therefore, having to a certain extent recruited her strength, she went to London, and took up her residence in Harley Street. Here an attempt had been made to create a "Home," a Sanitorium for sick ladies, mostly belonging to the governess class. It had been mismanaged, and she found it most desolate and unhomelike. Here was work to her hand, and without hesitation she threw herself heart and soul into the re-organisation of the establishment, into bringing order and comfort into the house, and something like happiness and content into the weary lives of those who had spent themselves in fulfilling the most arduous, and as a rule the most thankless of missions, that of rearing other people's children, doing a mother's work, without either the love or gratitude which alone can make the task easy.

It would be out of place here to expatiate on the miseries of a governess's life. It is a recognised fact that it was the loneliest, most dreary existence a young girl, gently born and gently nurtured, could be condemned to lead. Cut off from her own people, from her own associates, she stood apart with no well-defined position in the household. To the servants the fact of her receiving remuneration placed her in their estimation on an equality with themselves—she remained always only the governess. She was outside the pale of the family circle, she was not expected to intrude upon it beyond what her duties necessitated, so that enforced isolation was the natural result, and this engenders acute sensitiveness. Then children, very charming to outsiders, are often difficult to manage, and so, what with the lack of sympathy and the continual friction of petty annoyances, a certain irritability and sense of injustice creeps over even the bravest hearts. It is an established fact that our female lunatic asylums, at the time of which we are writing, and for some years afterwards, reckoned more governesses among their inmates than members of any other class. By degrees this state of things has improved; there are more occupations open to women, public education is more general, and in the course of time probably the whole system of home education will be done away with. That exclusiveness which was, and still is, so marked a characteristic of English life, is yielding to the progressive spirit of the age. What we may call public education, even for girls, is the order of the day, and families who twenty or thirty years ago would have shrunk from the very idea of sending their children to school or abroad, do not hesitate now. The result, of course, is a marked improvement in the education of the girls in the upper class of society; the governesses themselves are more fitted for their tasks, their minds are more developed, they have a wider knowledge of men and things, and they are more independent. But now, as then, they are not an enviable class, and with her large philanthropy Florence Nightingale felt this evil, and brought all her loving sympathy, all her newly acquired knowledge, to help in the work which had been attempted to make a home for these sad and lonely ones in the world. "Ye have the poor always with you," they are easy to find, but these solitary embittered souls have to be *sought* out.

It needed a tender touch and great patience to bring balm to wounds in which the arrows of neglect still rankled, to soothe false pride, to bear with the daily bickerings, to sit by the dying bed and tell of a better and happier world, where disappointed hopes would blossom into flowers. All this she did and much more of which there is no record, save on the tablets of the recording angel. She organised and brought order and comfort where previously little of either had existed, but above all things she sought to create a feeling of love and union. There was something in the fact of her having come to them of her own free will, which must have touched those sad hearts so little accustomed to be thought of—for them she had forsaken her beautiful home during the bright summer months to dwell in hot murky London, she shared the darkness and dullness of their long winter days, eschewing all the social pleasures to which her rank in society and her education gave her access, to make a home for the homeless, to share and if possible lessen their sorrows. And so from early morning till late at night she laboured at her self-imposed task, and the dull house in Harley Street was brightened by the sunshine of her gentle presence;

order was restored and harmony maintained.* She infused her own spirit into others, teaching the divine doctrine "to bear each others' burdens" by deeds of loving kindness.

But alas! the continual demands made on her, the mental strain, proved too much for Florence Nightingale's strength, and, however unwillingly, she was obliged to relinquish her post. Her physician ordered her entire rest, physical and mental, and so she once more turned her face homewards, and in the midst of dear friends, surrounded by all the associations of her happy childhood and girlhood, she settled down to recruit her failing powers. But not for one moment did she allow herself to forget the business of her life. She knew how to abide in patience, waiting quietly, until the path should of itself open out before her.

So Florence Nightingale breathed in the fresh air sweeping over the Derbyshire hills, and rejoiced with her presence the hearts of those who loved her, never dreaming that the day was near at hand when she must be up and doing. No, not even when the rumour of war filled the air, and the sound of battle reached her in her quiet home, did she know that her time of waiting was ended, that her powers were about to be tested to the uttermost, her noviciate was over.

* For this hospital she always retained an interest that never flagged. The lease expired a short time before her death, and a new site had to be acquired. The City of London had just conferred upon her the freedom of the City, and she begged the Lord Mayor to bestow on this little hospital the fifty pounds which would otherwise have been expended on the gold casket to contain the document. It was done as she desired, and in due course of time King George (then Prince of Wales) opened the hospital.

CHAPTER IV.

"FOR QUEEN AND COUNTRY."

"Three fishers went sailing out into the west,
 Out into the west, as the sun went down ;
Each thought of the woman who loved him best,
 And the children stood watching them out of the town ;
For men must work and women must weep,
For there's little to earn and many to keep,
 Though the harbour bar be moaning."

"PEACE on earth!" Only those who have experienced the horrors of war can truly realise the full significance and value of those three words.

To rise up in the morning and to lie down at night without fear in the quiet home with our dear ones around us, subject only to those ills which we cannot ward off; or to lie awake and think of the grim battlefield, the dead, the dying, the piteous moans of pain—ah, the contrast is so great, no marvel if we pray for peace!

For forty years England had been at rest, there was no call to war; the land prospered, commerce, the arts, and sciences flourished, wealth flowed in on every side, education and religion made rapid strides. The rival countries of England and France forgot old animosities, and extended to each other the hand of friendship. International exhibitions, marvellous for their wealth and beauty, united nations by one common bond, the peaceful arts; a sense of security pervaded the hearts of men, more especially in England. Other countries witnessed changes, thrones were overthrown, governments changed, but in our island, since Queen Victoria in her fair girlhood ascended the throne, there had been no disloyal thought; once only when there was a semblance of rebellion the gentry armed themselves to defend their queen and her laws. She reigned, honoured as a wife and mother—a shining light to every household.

It was in the midst of a peace such as this, in the year 1853, that a cloud arose in the east. When first visible it was no larger than a man's hand, and people smiled at the rumour of a possible war ; it was talked of vaguely, without exciting any real alarm. Our great warrior Wellington had but lately departed from amongst us, and been buried with such state and honour as had never before been accorded to an English soldier. Old things had passed away, and since the last European war, which had ended in the downfall of Napoleon, a new generation had sprung up, a new order of things reigned. If there was to be war it would differ materially from any previous warfare. Inventions had multiplied, the implements of war had changed. Upon the sea England had ever been great, but now she stood the unrivalled mistress of the seas. The harvest was gathered in, the autumn leaves lay upon the ground and were swept away by the north wind, snow

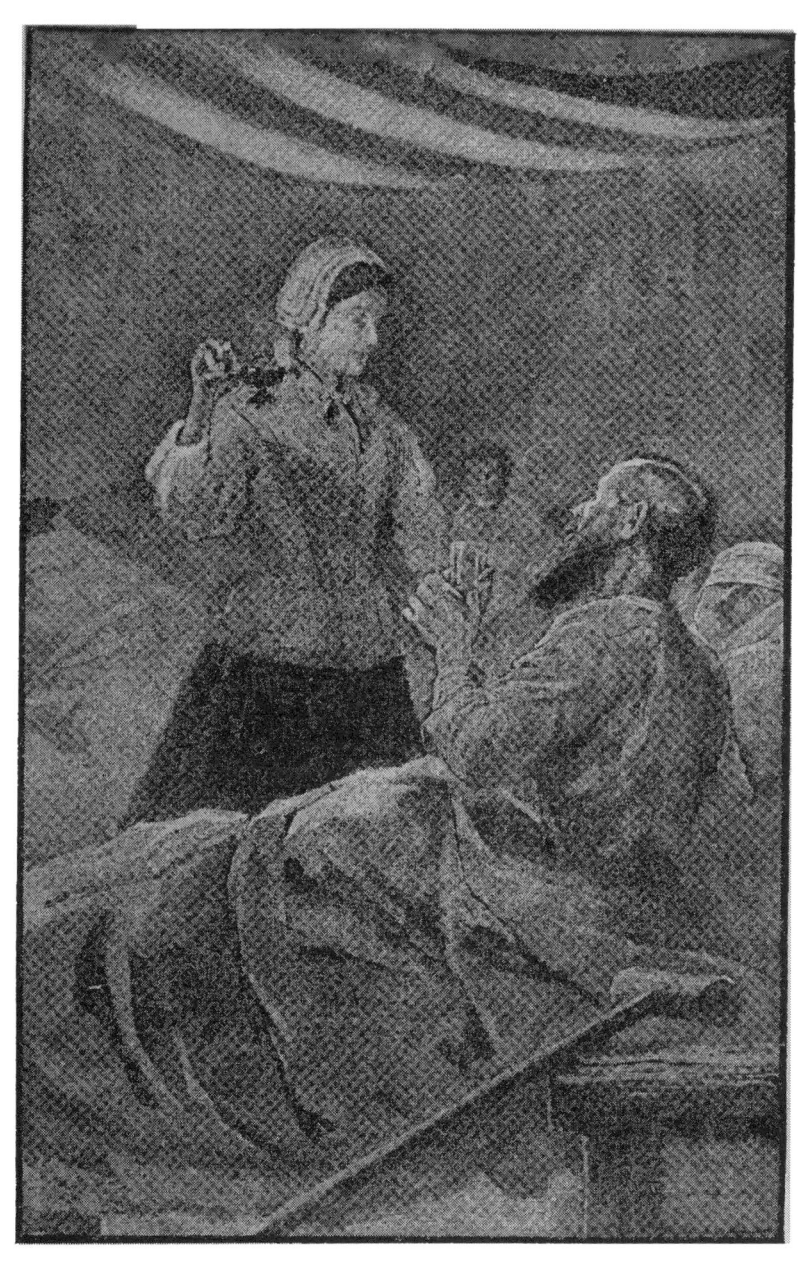

"THE LADY WITH THE LAMP."
Florence Nightingale making night visits to her Patients.

covered the earth, and the rumour became a growing certainty. Fathers looked proudly at their sons, and mothers trembled and hoped and prayed that the fear which haunted them by day and by night might pass away. A strange agitation vibrated throughout the length and breadth of England. Was it to be war or peace? Would Russia hear reason, or would she encroach upon the rights of others, and tread under her heel all principles of humanity and justice? If so, England must arise to strengthen the weak and the oppressed, she must throw the weight of her sword into the scales on the side of justice, and France elected to do likewise. Nevertheless those who stood at the helm strove to maintain peace, knowing only too well what the character of such a war would necessarily be. The vast resources of Russia, her immense army, the nature of her natural defences, and the unscrupulousness of her government, of all this and much more they were aware; therefore by every means in their power the allies sought to avoid war, but in vain—the science of diplomacy failed, and as the old year drew to a close the fleets of France and England moved nearer and nearer the Black Sea, and on the 30th of December sailed upon its dark, troubled waters. Quietly and silently they took up their station, there was no declaration of war, they were ready to retire as rapidly as they had come if the enemy would do so likewise, but as long as the Russians held the Danubian provinces, so long would they manifest their disapprobation by their presence in the Bosphorus. And so the year 1853 came to a close; it was an unusually severe winter, and the snow lay thick upon the ground; many a sad heart, filled with forebodings, must have watched the old year die out and the dawn of the new. Eighteen hundred and fifty four! what would it bring forth? would some of England's noblest sons be laid low for her honour's sake? None could tell. They were ready and willing to obey her call; whatever the arguments, and they were numerous, brought forward in favour of the war, they were almost unanimously accepted by the English people.

As the days and weeks slipped by, so all hope of peace passed away. Russia proved inexorable, France and England had stated through their ambassadors the terms upon which they were willing to maintain peace, and no further discussion was possible. The preparations for war were actively pursued. Little more than fifty years previously, on the 12th of March, 1801, an English fleet had set sail for the Baltic, under the command of Lord Nelson. In the year of our Lord, 1854, in the same month of March, almost on the same day, another English fleet, in the command of Admiral Sir Charles Napier, stood off Spithead, waiting for the Queen of England to come and bid them "God speed" ere they put out to sea, bound for the same destination.

Gloriously, we are told, the sun shone forth that day on the dancing waters, covered with ships of every dimension, from the mighty men-of-war to the light yacht cruising hither and thither. Suddenly from the flag-staff ship the boom of a gun broke over the waters, and instantly the beautiful royal yacht the *Fairy*, having the Queen on board, steamed through the line of men-of-war, each ship manning the rigging, and cheering heartily as she passed by. Then the admirals and the captains, in obedience to the royal command, went on board the *Fairy* to take personal leave of Her Majesty. To each she spoke a few words of farewell, and, after shaking hands with Sir Charles, "it was observed," we are told, "that she was affected to tears." Then each commander returned to his own ship, and the order was given, "Put out to sea." We read of ancient sea legends, of Salamis, of Cleopatra at the head of her fleet, and we picture to ourselves the grandeur of those ancient times, when perhaps history never recorded a more touching and imposing sight than was witnessed when the English fleet started on this bright March morning for the Baltic. It may not be amiss to give the description in the words of an eyewitness, at least it will be more graphic, warmer of colouring. It is thus told :—

"The operation of weighing and making sail was performed by the flag-ship with admirable celerity and precision. Every rope was hauled home in a moment by the silent and simultaneous effort of a hundred men, the rigging was soon black with sailors, and while the eye detected everywhere the greatest energy and activity, to the ear there was no sound perceptible but the boatswain's whistle and an occasional command from an officer, sharp, short, and decisive. The *Fairy* now shot past, heading the fleet, Her Majesty literally leading them out to sea, standing on deck all the time, and watching every movement with an interest which never tired.

"When did ever British sailors have such incentives to deeds of daring—led thus almost into action by the foremost lady in the world, to be defenders at once of her woman's helplessness and her royal honour? 'Truth is stranger than fiction,' and never did poet or dramatist imagine so fine a situation as that afforded by the stern realities of the departure of the Baltic fleet. Within a mile of the Nab the *Fairy* hove to, and then the whole fleet sailed by, driven out to sea by a beautiful west breeze. 'Her Majesty,' we are told, 'stood waving her handkerchief, as the mighty flag-ship, with the admiral on board, passed by, and for a long time after the whole fleet had gone the royal yacht remained motionless, as if the illustrious occupant desired to linger over the impressive spectacle.' The fleet was gone, carrying with it the prayers of a whole nation, and the Queen returned to Osborne, as many a wife and sweetheart returned to their humbler homes, with trembling lips and tearful eyes, repeating sadly, yet proudly, 'England expects every man to do his duty.'"

Before the end of the same month the declaration of war was formally made and the ambassadors of France and England withdrew from the Russian capital. The certainty that war was now inevitable entered every heart, even into those who to the eleventh hour had entertained the hope that peace might still be possible. Very various must have been the feelings it brought into play, every human sensibility, which for fifty years had lain dormant, awoke—ambition, aspirations, visions of high honours for the actors in the approaching warfare. Many a heart aches for those who staying at home remembered sadly the poet's words—" The path of glory leads but to the grave." How many a home would in the course of the next few months realize the truth of these words? How many a fair young life would have its earthly career with all its bright hopes cut short! Europe was suddenly

Leopard, Edinburgh, Princess Royal, D. of Wellington, Tribune, Royal George, Blenheim, Ajax, Fairy, Arrogant, Hogue, Jean D'Acre, Impérieuse, Amphion

BALTIC FLEET LEAVING SPITHEAD.

transformed into two vast camps, about to fight it
out, until moderation should be taught to the proud,
or submission forced upon the weak. Throughout
the length and breadth of England there was from
henceforth but one subject of conversation—the war!
All eyes were turned towards those armies manœuvr-
ing on the "swampy flats of the lower Danube," or
upon the stately fleet steaming to unknown perils
over a bleak, unfamiliar sea.

Very characteristic was Sir Charles Napier's
announcement, made by signal to the fleet lying at
anchor in Kioge Bay :—

"Lads, war is declared. We are to meet a bold
and numerous enemy. Should they offer us battle,
you know how to dispose of them. Should they
remain in port, we must try to get at them. Success
depends upon the quickness and decision of your fire.
Lads sharpen your cutlasses and the day is ours."

Need we say that such words were received with
enthusiastic cheering? And so, in the bright spring
sunshine and in the early summer, preparations went
on with stirring rapidity.

The English Generals follow the French Generals
to the scene of action—the dispatch of troops, the
departure of officers, the launching of ships, such were
the sole topics of the day.

For the first time in history France and England
had fraternised, and their soldiers were about to fight
side by side in a common cause. People shook their
heads. Was it possible, they asked, that thus suddenly
the animosity of centuries should be laid on one
side? That two proverbially hostile nations should
extend to each other the hand of fellowship? Could
the French forget Waterloo?

E

To their eternal honour let it be recorded that if they did not forget, they bore no malice, but during those many months of warfare fought bravely side by side with our own soldiers, performing unrivalled deeds of valour, and proving themselves our true allies, not only on the battlefield, but in the hospital, beneath the tent, as in the trenches, before Sebastopol.

Following upon the declaration of war, in the midst of the din and excitement, the order came calm and clear, stilling all worldly passions, bidding hearts throbbing with pain or elated with the anticipation of glory to be still, "Let my people hold a fast day to the Lord." And in all humility the nation acquiesced ; before sending its armies out to battle it acknowledged the Divine Providence overruling all things. Never in the annals of the country was a fast so generally and so devoutly observed by all classes, and then, as if comforted, each went their way to await in patience the result. As the summer months sped by the fear of pestilence was added to the growing horrors of war ; it was a terrible time, and the lingering uncertainty tried the bravest hearts.

Suddenly there was a shout of victory. Alma had been fought and won, followed quickly by the equally glorious day of Inkerman ; and then across the water came a cry for help, the sick and wounded were lying uncared for, many were dying because there was none to tend them. "Where are our women? will not they help us as only women can, with their tender touch and their gentle presence? surely they will not leave us to die like dogs, they will come to us." And the call was answered wisely and well, not with a wild enthusiastic zeal, though there was no lack of enthusiasm, but with head and hand as well as heart, without which the results must have been very different from what they turned out. One who has gone to his rest, beloved and revered of all, Mr. Sydney Herbert, stood at the helm, and with steady hand and sure eye directed the movement, and did much towards its success.

CHAPTER V

"THE CALL."

"And happy they who none deplore,
Laid low beside the Black Sea shore,
Whom white-robed peace shall bring no more
    To swell her smiling train !
Peace be with those who must their loss deplore,
    And honour to the slain."

THE great battle of Alma was fought and won, and though as a country we rejoiced, individually there was much sorrow for those who would "never come back again." Then the rumour spread rapidly that the sanitary administration had broken down, and that our men were dying from neglect and misery. A letter from William Howard Russell, *The Times* correspondent, raised the public indignation to fever heat. The letter ran thus :—

"The commonest accessories of a hospital are wanting; there is not the least attention paid to decency or cleanliness, the stench is appalling; the fœtid air can barely struggle out to taint the atmosphere, save through the chinks in the walls and roofs ;

and for all I can observe, the men die without the least effort being made to save them.

"There they lie just as they were let gently down on the ground by the poor fellows, their comrades, who brought them on their backs from the camp, with the greatest tenderness, but who are not allowed to remain with them.

"The sick appear to be tended by the sick, and the dying by the dying."

And this was followed by an appeal which touched all hearts.

"Are there no devoted women amongst us, able and willing to go forth to minister to the sick and suffering soldiers of the East in the hospitals of Scutari? Are none of the daughters of England, at this extreme hour of need, ready for such a work of mercy?

"France has sent forth her sisters of mercy unsparingly, and they are even now by the bedsides of the wounded and the dying, giving what woman's hand alone can give of comfort and relief in such awful scenes of suffering.

"Our soldiers have fought beside the troops of France, certainly with no inferior courage and devotedness, in one of the most sanguinary and terrific battles ever recorded.

"Must we fall so far below the French in self-sacrifice and devotedness, in a work which Christ so signally blesses as done unto Himself? 'I was sick and ye visited Me.'"

It is not to be supposed that such a call would remain long unanswered. Other appeals followed— an officer's wife who had gone out with her husband writes:

"Oh what a terrible time this is! Could you see the scenes that we are daily witnessing, you would indeed be distressed. I am still in barracks, but the sick are now lying in the passages, within a few yards of my room. Every corner is being filled up with the sick and wounded. However, I am enabled to do some little good, and I hope I shall not be obliged to leave just yet. My time is occupied in cooking for the wounded. Three doors from me there is an officer's wife who devotes herself to cooking for the sick. There are no female nurses here, which decidedly there ought to be. The French have sent fifty sisters of mercy who, we need hardly say, are devoted to the work. We are glad to hear that some efforts are being made at home. The master of St. John's Home, the training institution for nurses at Westminster, states, 'that a body of nurses, as many as can be spared, are about to be sent immediately from the Institution.'"

Worse accounts followed, harrowing even to those who had no loved ones among the sufferers. What then must have been the feelings of mothers and sisters and sweethearts? One account of the poor wounded soldiers' voyage across the water to Scutari, unattended by any medical men, excited the greatest indignation. "On their arrival," it said, "they found no preparation for the commonest surgical operations; the commonest appliances of a workhouse sick ward were wanting, and the men must die through the medical staff of the British army having forgotten that old rags are necessary for the dressing of wounds."

Of course, in this account allowances must be made for exaggeration and excited feelings; the

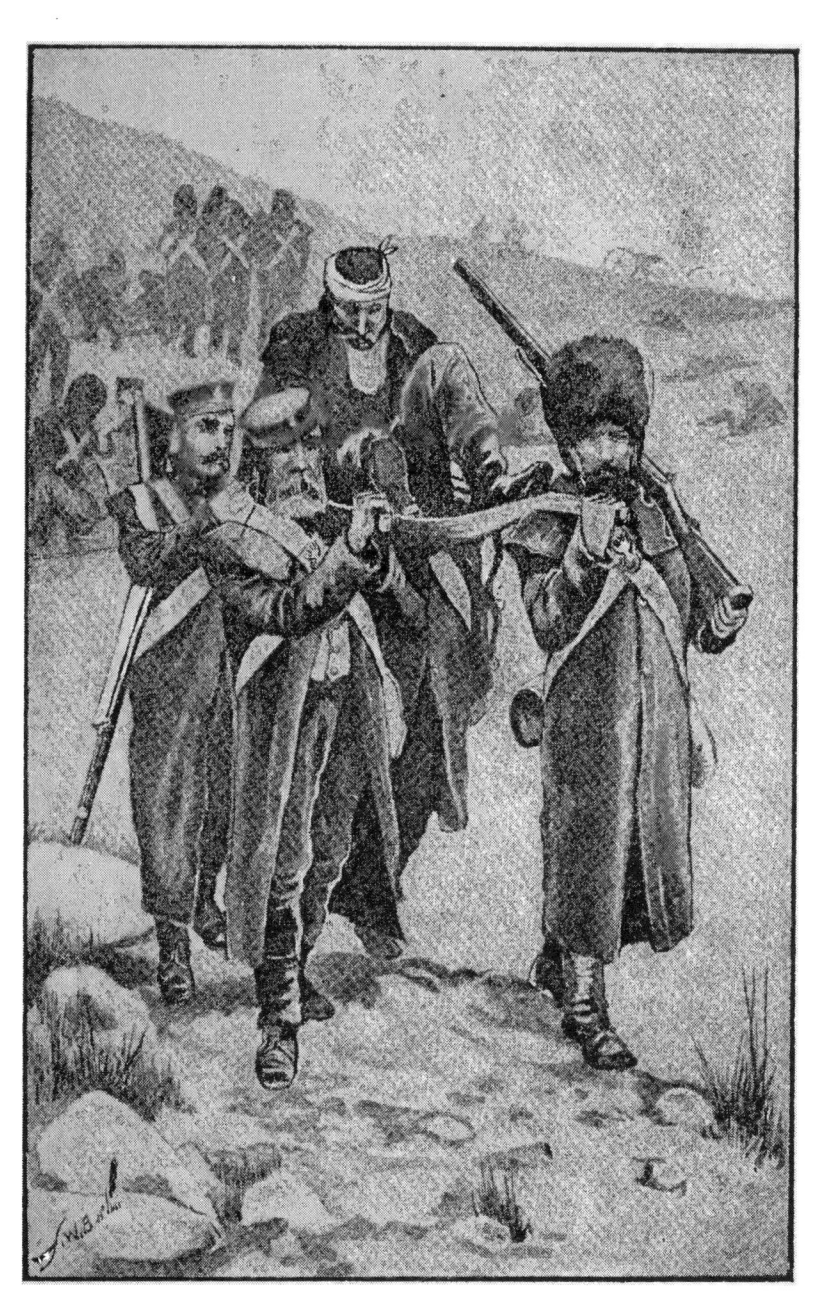

GUARDS CARRYING WOUNDED OFFICER.

result, however, was magical. Sir Robert Peel wrote to the *Times* enclosing a cheque for two hundred pounds, and in the course of *one* day the *Times* received two thousand pounds. But though money was a welcome accessory, it was not *the* thing. An enthusiastic desire to answer the appeal was felt throughout England. But inexperienced zeal could perform little, and a bevy of ill-organised nurses might do more harm than good. There was a fear lest a noble impulse should fail for the want of a head, a hand, and a heart to direct it. But there was one who in the quiet seclusion of her beautiful Derbyshire home heard and pondered over these things. She knew her own power, she understood now, perhaps for the first time, the end and object of those long years of patient training. As she paced slowly, in those early October days, beneath the avenue of beech trees, just tinted with the golden hues of autumn, she thought of her countrymen dying far away with none to help them. Men in their high heroism might dash up the heights of Alma, but woman alone could bring her power of consolation, her ready help and her loving sympathy, to ease the rack-tortured body, and smooth the dying pillow. She knew what was needed, and she knew, too, that she was capable of answering to the full that bitter cry for help which had come wafted across the seas.

It was not in her nature to hesitate; those who loved her best attempted no word of opposition, they had long since recognised her mission as one of "God's ministering angels upon earth."

On the 15th of October, little more than a fortnight after the battle of Alma, quietly, as it was her wont to do everything, Florence Nightingale sat down and wrote to Mr. Sidney Herbert, then Minister of War, offering her services as nurse to the army in the East. But, silently as she had lived, her value was well known by those most capable of appreciating it. The same day on which she posted

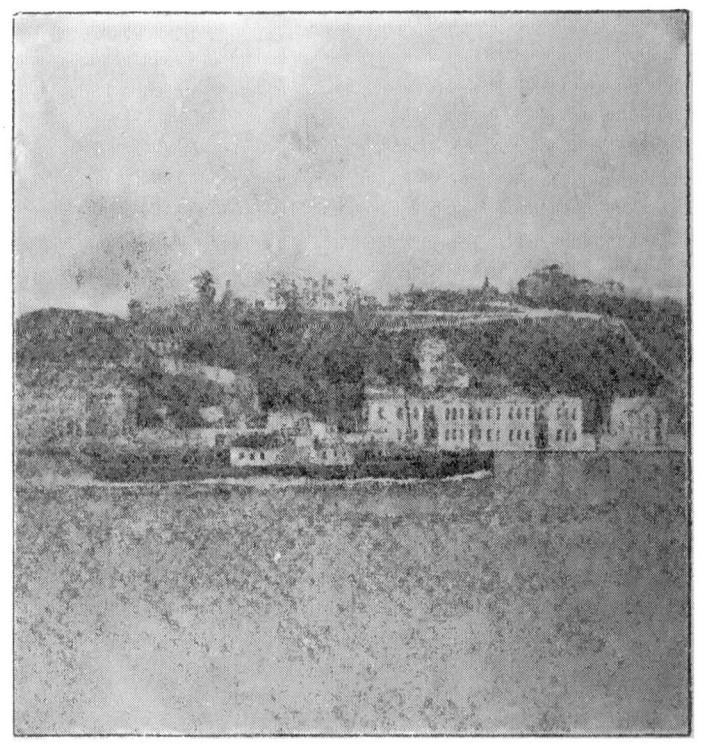

VIEW OF THE BOSPHORUS, SHOWING THE HOSPITAL AT SCUTARI.

her offer to help, he had written her the following letter. The two epistles crossed each other.

"Dear Miss Nightingale,—You will have seen in the papers that there is a great deficiency of nurses at the hospital of Scutari. The other alleged deficiencies, namely, of medical men, lint sheets, etc., must, if they ever existed, have been remedied ere this, as the number of medical officers with the army amounted to one to every ninety-five men in the whole force, being nearly double what we have ever had before; and thirty more surgeons went out there three weeks ago, and must by this time, therefore, be at Constantinople. A further supply went on Monday, and a fresh batch sail next week. As to medical stores, they have been sent out in profusion, by the ton weight—15,000 pair of sheets, medicine, wine, arrowroot in the same proportion, and the only way of accounting for the deficiency at Scutari, if it exists, is that the mass of the stores went to Varna, and had not been sent back when the army left for the Crimea, but four days would have remedied that.

"In the meanwhile, stores are arriving, but the deficiency of female nurses is undoubted; none but male nurses have ever been admitted to military hospitals. It would be impossible to carry about a large staff of female nurses with an army in the field. But at Scutari, having now a fixed hospital, no military reason exists against the introduction, and I am confident they might be introduced with great benefit, for hospital orderlies must be very rough hands, and most of them, on such an occasion at this, very inexperienced ones. I receive numbers of offers from ladies to go out, but they are ladies who have no conception of what an hospital is, nor of the nature of its duties; and they would, when the time came, either recoil from the work or be entirely useless, and consequently, what is worse, entirely in the way; nor would those ladies probably even understand the necessity, especially in a military hospital, of strict obedience to rule, etc.

"Lady Maria Forrester (Lord Roden's daughter) has made some proposal to Dr. Smith, the head of the army medical department, either to go with, or to send out trained nurses.

"I apprehend she means from Fitzroy Square, John Street, or some such establishment. The Rev. Mr. Hume, once chaplain to the general hospital at Birmingham (and better known as the author of the scheme for transferring the city churches to the suburbs), has offered to go out himself, as chaplain, with two daughters and twelve nurses. He was in the army seven years and has been used to hospitals, and I like the tone of his letter very much. I think from both these offers practical effects may be drawn. But the difficulty of finding nurses who are at all versed in their business is probably best known to Mr. Hume, and Lady Maria Forrester has not tested the willingness of the trained nurses to go, and is incapable of directing or ruling them. There is but one person in England that I know of, who would be capable of organising and superintending such a scheme, and I have been several times on the point of asking you hypothetically if, supposing the attempt were made, you would undertake to direct it. The selection of the rank and file of nurses would be difficult, no one knows that better than yourself. The difficulty of finding women equal to a task after all full of horror, and requiring, besides knowledge and good-will, great knowledge and great courage, will be great; the task of ruling them and introducing system among them, great; and not the least will be the difficulty of making the whole work smoothly with the

"THE CALL." 77

medical and military authorities out there. This it is
which makes it so important that the experiment
should be carried out by one with administrative
capacity and experience. A number of sentimental,
enthusiastic ladies turned loose in the hospital at
Scutari would probably, after a few days, be *mises
à la porte*, by those whose business they would
interrupt, and whose authority they would dispute.
My question simply is, would you listen to the request
to go out and supervise the whole thing? You would,
of course, have plenary authority over all the nurses,
and I think I could secure you the fullest assistance
and co-operation from the medical staff, and you
would also have an unlimited power of drawing on the
Government for whatever you think requisite for the
success of your mission. On this part of the subject
the details are too many for a letter, and I reserve it
for our meeting; for, whatever decision you take,
I know you will give me every assistance and advice.
I do not say one word to press you. You are the
only person who can judge for yourself which of con-
flicting or incompatible duties is the first or the highest; but I think I must not conceal from you that
upon your decision will depend the ultimate success or
failure of the plan. Your own personal qualities, your
knowledge, and your power of administration, and,
among greater things, your rank and position in
society, give you advantages in such a work which no
other person possesses. If this succeeds an enormous
amount of good will be done now, and to persons
deserving everything at our hands; and which will
multiply the good to all time. I hardly like to be
sanguine as to your answer. If it were yes, I am
certain the Bracebridges would go with you, and give

you all the comforts you would require, and which her society and sympathy only could give you. I have written very long, for the subject is very near my heart. Liz is writing to our mutual friend, Mrs. Bracebridge, to tell her what I am doing. I go back to town to-morrow morning. Shall I come to you between three and five? Will you let me have a line at the War Office, to let me know? There is one point which I have hardly a right to touch upon, but I trust you will pardon me. If you were inclined to undertake the great work, would Mr. and Mrs. Nightingale consent? This work would be so national, and the request made to you, proceeding from the Government which represents the nation, comes at such a moment that I do not despair of their consent. Deriving your authority from the Government, your position would ensure the respect and consideration of every one, especially in a service where official rank carries so much weight. This would secure you any attention or comfort on your way out there, together with a complete submission to your orders. I know these things are a matter of indifference to you, except as far as they may further the great object you may have in view; but they are of importance in themselves, and of every importance to those who have a right to take an interest in your personal position and comfort. I know you will come to a right and wise decision. God grant it may be one in accordance with my hopes.—Believe me, Dear Miss Nightingale, ever yours,

"SIDNEY HERBERT."

The quiet trust expressed throughout this letter in the wisdom and unselfishness of her to whom it was addressed, is the best proof we can have of the estimation in which Florence Nightingale was held by those who knew her most intimately. Throughout the whole of it the intense desire of the writer is apparent, kept under by the respect which he felt in her judgment. Coming from a man of such high standing, and so reverenced as was Mr. Sydney Herbert, any woman might have been flattered; and we may feel assured that as she read it a glad feeling must have come over her, with the certainty that she had not over-estimated her powers, that she was in very truth equal to the task which lay before her, that her instincts and her strong desires had not led her to overrate her capabilities. It must have been with a feeling almost of exultation that she remembered that at the same moment as she was reading his request, he, the Minister of War to whom everybody looked for help, was in receipt of her offer. She was glad she had not delayed, glad she had acted spontaneously, without counting the cost, as one who knows that she is the servant of God and that she has no right to withhold the gifts which are His, the talents He has bestowed. In her own mind the whole thing was settled, and from that hour nothing remained for her to do but to make her necessary preparations. It was, as Mr. Sydney Herbert had warned her, no easy task, more especially the choosing of nurses. Money flowed in; she neither asked nor refused pecuniary aid. All subscriptions were to be paid into Messrs. Coutts' bank to her account.

In the course of the next few days all England was ringing with her name. "Who was Miss Nightingale?" the papers asked, and even ventured to sneer at the idea of "a young, unmarried lady" going out as hospital nurse; but whilst she herself kept silence, occupied only in the preparations necessary for the carrying out of her self-imposed task, others, jealous of her honour, answered for her. A portion of an article published in the *Examiner* is not devoid of interest, and may fitly find its place here. "Who is Mrs. Nightingale? Many ask this question, and it has not yet been adequately answered. We reply then: Mrs. Nightingale is Miss Nightingale, or rather Miss Florence Nightingale, the youngest daughter, and presumptive co-heiress of her father, William Shore Nightingale of Embley Park, Hampshire, and Lea Hurst, Derbyshire. She is, moreover, a lady of singular endowments, both natural and acquired. In the knowledge of the ancient languages and of the higher branches of mathematics, in general science and literature, her attainments are extraordinary. There is scarcely a modern language which she does not understand, and she speaks German, French, and Italian as fluently as her native English. She has visited and studied the various nations of Europe, and has ascended the Nile to its remotest cataract. Young (about the age of our Queen), graceful, feminine, rich, and popular, she holds a singularly gentle and persuasive influence over all with whom she comes in contact. Her friends and acquaintances are of all classes and persuasions, but her happiest place is at home, in the centre of a very large band of accomplished relatives, and in simplest obedience to admiring parents. Why then should a being so highly blessed with all that should render life bright, innocent, and, to a considerable extent, useful, forego such palpable and heartfelt attractions? Why quit all this to become a nurse?" Then a slight sketch was given of her young life, "her yearning affection for her kind, her sympathy with the weak, the sick the destitute. The life of training to which she had voluntarily submitted," and the article wound up with these pathetic words:—

"A sage few will no doubt condemn, sneer at, or pity an enthusiasm which to them seems eccentric or at best misplaced ; but to the true heart of the country it will speak home, and by it be felt that there is not one of England's proudest and purest daughters who at this moment stands on so high a pinnacle as Florence Nightingale."

CHAPTER VI.

"AT THE HELM."

> "O woman! in our hours of ease,
> Uncertain, coy, and hard to please,
> And variable as the shade
> By the light quivering aspen made;
> When pain and anguish wring the brow,
> A ministering angel thou."

FROM morning till late at night, Miss Nightingale laboured to organise her staff of nurses. Party spirit ran high, every one discussed this simple, earnest, Christian woman. With one set she was a Papist, with another a Dissenter! It is doubtful whether she was herself aware of the *on dits* which filled the papers.

But both she and her faithful friends, Mr. and Mrs. Sydney Herbert, were overwhelmed with letters, applications, and the necessity of interviewing those who applied to be admitted on her staff of nurses. She had intended to leave England on the 17th of October, but for these and other reasons was obliged to delay a few days. She named two other ladies to assist her in the selection of nurses, whose first step was to advertise in the *Record* and *Guardian*. Miss Nightingale applied to the known institutions. In the meantime Roman Catholic bishops and private individuals wrote to the War Office, offering to go out to the East taking nurses with them. No definite answer was given until Miss Nightingale's appointment was announced, giving her full authority to form her own band, that band being subject to her in all matters relating to the hospital. Submission was the first and primary law laid down. The nurses belonging to one or two institutions would not consent to go under such conditions. The Roman Catholic bishop agreed at once to these terms, and signed a paper to that effect. Rules were issued to the Sisters of Mercy for this especial service, the first of which was that the Sisters should attend to the corporal and spiritual wants of the Roman Catholic soldiers, and that they should never enter into discussion or controversy with any but those of their own faith. St. John's House demurred to the severance from their own society and complete submission to Miss Nightingale, but after two or three days' consideration they accepted. It was the same with other institutions, but by degrees, several sent in their adhesion. By Saturday the 21st of October, just a week after she had made her offer of help, Florence Nightingale's band was completed.

10 Roman Catholic Sisters of Mercy,
 8 Of Miss Sellon's,
 6 From St. John's House,
 3 Selected by the lady who commenced the plan,
11 Selected among applicants.

On the same day Mr. Herbert announced from the War Office that Miss Nightingale and her staff of 38 nurses would start that evening for Scutari. They were to sail on the 26th from Marseilles for Constantinople in the *Vectis*, a fast steamer of the Peninsular Company, employed usually in the carriage of the Indian Mail, and were expected to reach their destination about the 4th of November. Mr. and Mrs. Bracebridge accompanied Miss Nightingale, also a clergyman and a courier.

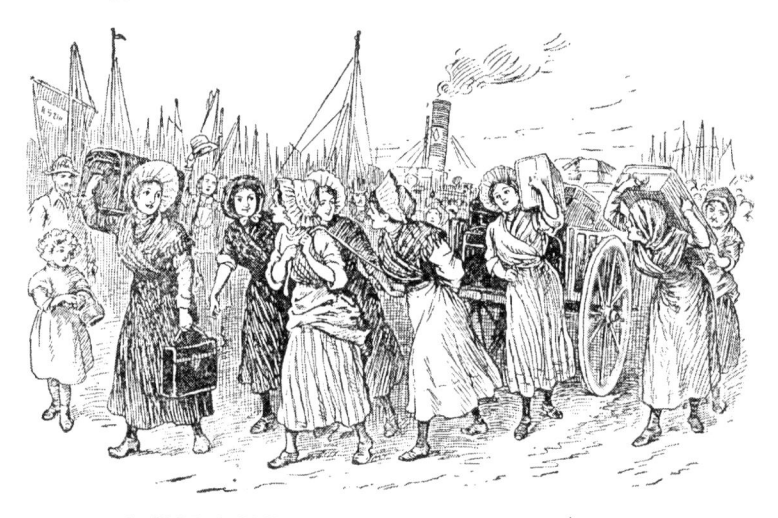

BOULOGNE FISHERWOMEN CARRYING NURSES' BAGGAGE.

Very quietly under cover of night that devoted band left London. Above everything they were desirous of avoiding public observation. "Let not thy right hand know what thy left hand doeth," but they were not entirely successful in this. When they landed at Boulogne a rumour had got abroad among the fisherwomen, who act as porters, that a band of English

Sisters were on their way to the Crimea to nurse the sick and wounded. Nothing was likely to appeal so forcibly to the French nature, especially to this class, as the fact that their soldiers were to be cared for and tended. There is not a household in France in which one or two at least of its members are not *sous les drapeaux*, and when in the early morning the steam packet with the nurses on board entered the Boulogne Harbour, the *quai* was crowded with brawny fisher-women, young and old, in crimson petticoats, with many-coloured kerchiefs folded across their bosoms, and with their large plaited snowy caps, and long gold earrings; they stood there eager, not noticing the ordinary passengers, only waiting for *les sœurs*, and when the quiet band in their black cloaks appeared, there was a rush forward. It was who should carry their bags, their wraps, their trunks; they would have carried the Sisters themselves if they had not feared to offend! "Pay them! ah, no indeed, not a sou would they take, only if they would shake hands, and if they should happen to come across their Jacques, or their Pierre——" Poor souls! Many a tear was brushed away as the train steamed out of the station to the cry of *vive les sœurs*—God help them. Meantime her friends were fighting Miss Nightingale's battles at home; sad that there should have been any necessity for so doing, but alas, petty jealousy and narrow-minded bigotry are seldom lacking even in the holiest cause. Everything that could be said or written to quiet and satisfy the most susceptible was done. One statement is worth recording :—

"These are the plain facts of the case," says the writer. "No party feeling has had anything to do with the appointment of Miss Nightingale. There has not been a shade of rivalry between her and any one else. We are assured that there has been no desire on Mr. Sidney Herbert's part to favour Popery, either in the first selection of nurses or in the more recent arrangements. Those of the nurses who have been either Sisters of Mercy or Sisters of Charity cease—in the technical sense of the terms—to be so, by the footing on which they are gone out. They owe no obedience to any one but to Miss Nightingale.

"The Roman Catholic bishop has voluntarily, and in writing, released the benevolent persons who were previously under his control from all subjection to himself. Englishmen may have the pleasure of feeling that a number of kind-hearted British women, differing in faith but wishing to do practical good, are gone in one ship, as one corps, with one aim, without any compromise of our national Protestantism. Even the least Protestant of them must have felt, as they walked two and two under the guidance of Mr. and Mrs. Bracebridge round the scenes and sights of Malta, that the garb of an order or the shibboleth of a sect is not the divine method of uniting hearts.

"Thirty-eight nurses on their way to Scutari are truer successors of the Apostles shipwrecked at Melita, than an equal number of Cardinals. May the war teach men many such lessons!"

It was the 31st of October when the *Vectis* touched at Malta; it steamed off the same evening for Scutari, so anxious were those on board to reach their destination. One battle had been fought, and another was pending; they knew, therefore, that they would be needed. At last on the 5th of November they entered the Bosphorus and saw before them the "Silver City of Scutari" shining, as it is described,

"AT THE HELM." 87

"like a pearl," ten thousand feet above the dark troubled waters of the Black Sea. Scutari is regarded with great veneration by the Turks as being the place whence the founder of the Ottoman dynasty sprung. It was on the same day as the battle of Inkerman was fought that Miss Nightingale landed at Scutari,

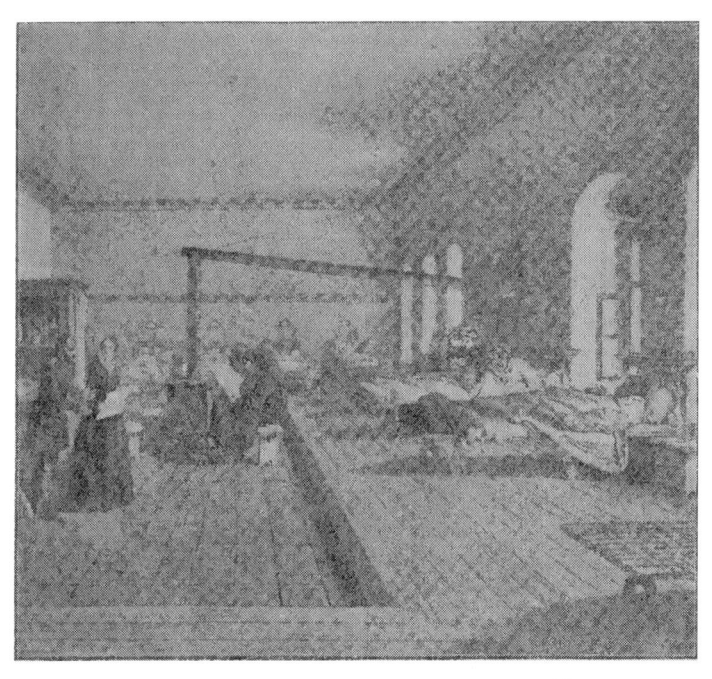

THE INTERIOR OF THE HOSPITAL AT SCUTARI—
FLORENCE NIGHTINGALE ON DUTY.

and she and her party were immediately comfortably lodged and provided for. In the afternoon we hear of some of them making their appearance on the shore, "cheerful and pleasant, neatly attired in black, a strong contrast to the usual aspect of hospital attendants, and oh, how welcome!"

They came none too soon, for in the course of the next few days 600 wounded were brought in from Inkerman. The surgeons, even the most prejudiced, could but confess that Miss Nightingale was the right woman in the right place. Her nerve was simply wonderful, her quiet systematic way of going to work, and organizing everything necessary for the care of the sick and wounded, inspired the clergy and medical men with a feeling of security. They had some one now to depend upon, and would from henceforth be spared the terrible sight of men sinking for want of proper nursing, and because food was not administered often enough. With the nurses, all that was needed was supplied. One poor fellow burst into tears, exclaiming, " I can't help it, I can't indeed, when I see them. Only think of English women coming out here to nurse us ; it is so homelike and comfortable."

Very quietly Florence Nightingale went about her work with such tact that she overcame, little by little, those who were most opposed to her. Her plan of action might almost have been said to be passive ; she supplied what was most urgently needed, interfering with no previous arrangements, she added to and filled up blanks in the administration. Her first act was to establish a sick kitchen where everything required in a sick-room was prepared with a quickness and nicety which the clumsy hospital arrangements rendered impossible. Sir Robert Peel's fund for the sick and wounded provided sago, arrowroot, wine, etc. The boon this kitchen was in special cases it is almost impossible now to realize. Besides this, from her quarters, without any of the formalities which application to Government entailed, wine,

"AT THE HELM." 89

brandy, clothes, could be procured at a minute's notice. When not engaged in nursing, the sisters were employed in arranging mattresses, making stump pillows for amputation cases; every imaginable comfort was procured from the Nightingale quarters. Her next act was to rent a laundry for the disinfecting and proper cleansing of the linen in the sick-wards, a matter of essential importance, as, unless linen for the wounded is thoroughly cleansed, it is apt to bring on erysipelas, and the hospital arrangements up to that time had been most unsatisfactory.

Nothing which could in any way help to smooth the sufferer's pillow, or aid the convalescent, was omitted by this wonderful woman, whose power of feeling was so great, it might almost have been thought she herself had borne the pain she sought so earnestly to ease. Wherever there was an omission she quietly stepped in to supply it, where there was a defect she sought unostentatiously to rectify it. Her greatest difficulty was to obtain Government stores; the amount of red tapeism to be gone through tried her patience sorely, as it did that of many others; and but for her firmness much of the stores and necessary surgical aid would not have been got at, at a season when they were most required. Once, even twice, she broke down the barriers which hemmed her in, and obtained by force of will for her sick soldiers the supplies which they stood so greatly in immediate need of.

Notwithstanding the appreciation which her services could not fail to meet with, the medical men, if they did not absolutely oppose, did little more than tolerate her. It was not till the end of December that Miss Nightingale and her nurses were regularly installed in the general hospital, where they had up to that time been, as I have said, merely tolerated, notwithstanding the work they did; a steady sort of tacit resistance was offered to their interference. The medical officers of the old routine could not be brought at once to comprehend that the great emergencies of the time had thus suddenly developed the female character and increased her influence. Protestant Germany had long ago her organized system of trained nurses, the order of St. Vincent de Paul in France was left unmolested even during the revolution, only in England it seemed incomprehensible to the general mind that ladies should take upon themselves a service which, until then, had been left in the hands of hirelings.

From early morning till late at night Florence Nightingale moved noiselessly hither and thither; the work she did was stupendous; not a report came before the public but her name was foremost in it. The chaplains, the clergy of all denominations spoke of her with reverence. "Miss Nightingale," one writes, "for that good woman takes brevet rank—is working her nurses admirably, being most judicious and excellent in all she does, and the sisters are of indescribable value!" She had to take everything into consideration, to refuse as well as to accept help, and her opinion was sought on all sides notwithstanding the jealousy to which she was subjected. But she walked steadily on from day to day doing her work as unto the Lord and not unto man. Several of the nurses she had brought with her had to be sent home, either through illness or incapacity, and their places had to be filled. Fresh detachments of nurses were sent out from England, one under Miss

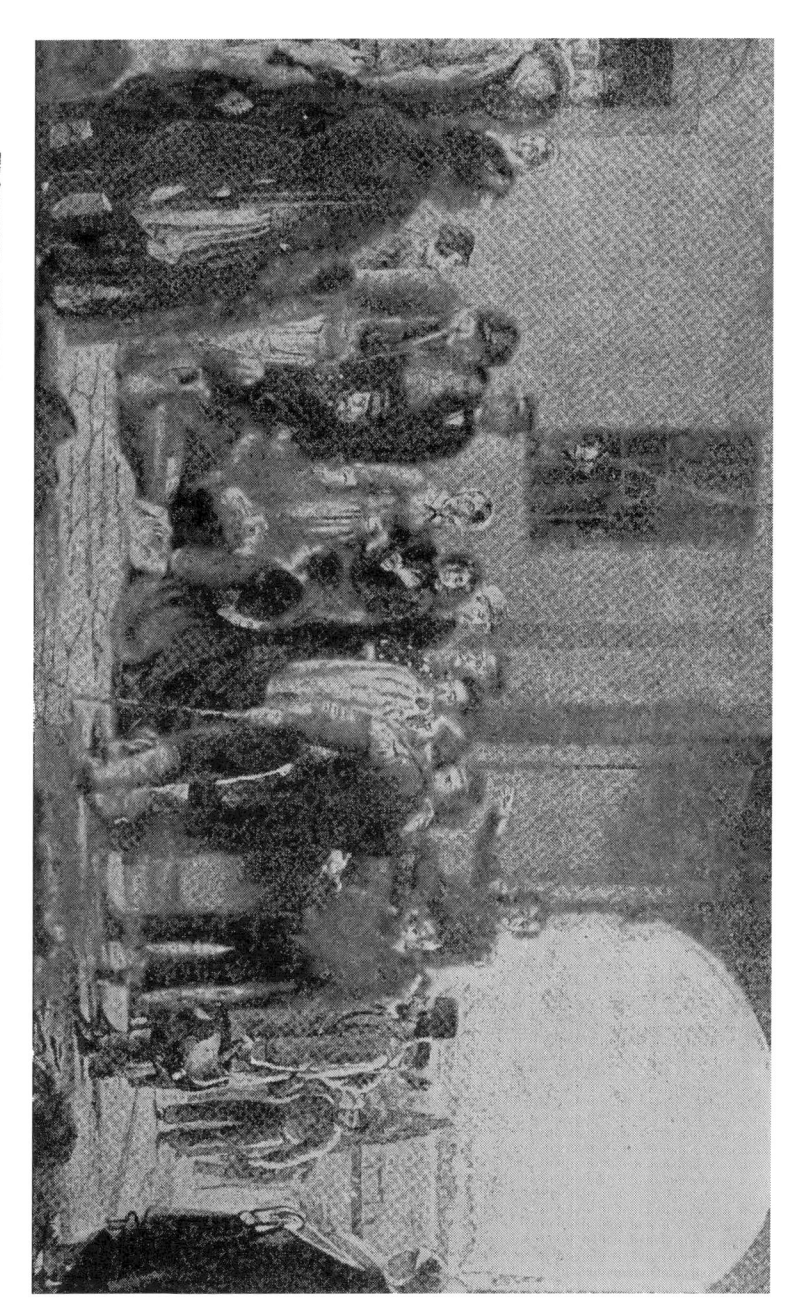

FLORENCE NIGHTINGALE RECEIVING WOUNDED SOLDIERS AT THE HOSPITAL AT SCUTARI.

"AT THE HELM." 93

Stanley for the working of other hospitals at Balaclava, Smyrna, Kululu, etc. The army suffered terribly, not only from wounds received in battle, but from frost-bites, dysentery, cholera, and many other ailments incident on exposure. The medical staff was also sorely tried. Mr. Macdonald the almoner of the *Times* writes very sadly :—

"At the Barrack Hospital there is hardly a single second class staff officer left. Dr. Summers is very ill, and Dr. Newton, I regret to say, is dead. Like poor Struthers, he too has fallen an untimely victim to the zeal with which he discharged his professional duties. It was fever of a low type in his case also ; and, indeed, it is so rife now in every direction, that the wonder is how more of the healthy and strong are not struck down by it. Both Newton and Struthers, it may be a consolation to their friends to know, were tended in their last moments and their eyes closed by Miss Nightingale herself."

What greater praise could be given to any woman than that it "must necessarily be a comfort" to the mourners that she should close the eyes of their "beloved." The aching mother's or wife's heart, wrung with anguish, was soothed by the thought that the place they would so gladly have occupied was not quite desolate, and that the departing souls went home with a woman's voice whispering a prayer, a woman's hand to close the dying eyes and straighten the weary limbs at their journey's end. Unceasingly the work went on ; and the name of Florence Nightingale in less than two months was a "household word," never to be forgotten. How she lived through that time she alone could tell, if she would ; but one thing is certain, it was not in her own strength that she accomplished her work, and she knew it. Her gracious presence in the sick wards brought comfort. "To see her pass is happiness," said a poor fellow writing home. "She would speak to one, and nod and smile to many more, but she could not do it to all, you know. We lay there by hundreds; but we could kiss her shadow as it fell, and lay our heads upon the pillow again content."

Can any tribute be more touchingly pathetic?

"So in that house of misery,
A lady with a lamp I see
  Pass through the glimmering gloom,
  And flit from room to room.

"And slowly, as in a dream of bliss,
The speechless sufferer turns to kiss
  Her shadow, as it falls
  Upon the darkening walls.

"On England's annals, through the long
Hereafter of her speech and song,
  A light its rays shall cast,
  From portals of the past.

"A lady with a lamp shall stand,
In the great history of the land,
  A noble type of good,
  Heroic Womanhood."

CHAPTER VII.

A MESSAGE.

> "But the good deed, through the ages
> Living in historic pages,
> Brighter glows and gleams immortal
> Unconsumed by moth or rust."

THOSE years of quiet preparation brought forth their fruit now; the knowledge Miss Nightingale had acquired, and was able to make practical use of, astonished all who came in contact with her.

Her skill was so considerable, that more than one medical man has asserted that she surpassed many men in both theoretical and practical knowledge. Among the labours of Hercules is numbered as not the least arduous the cleansing of the Augean stables; a very similar task fell to the lot of this delicately-reared lady.

Round the hospital the greatest uncleanliness existed—Miss Nightingale herself counted in one day six dogs in a state of decomposition lying under the hospital windows. This was enough alone to engender fever, but when we consider that the water was impure and that many other abuses existed, we can scarcely be surprised at the frightful rate of mortality. So ill-kept and crowded was the hospital that we are told, "the sufferers, to add to their other miseries, were tormented by vermin, and that the rats attacked the limbs of those who were too weak to defend themselves." The meals were a simple pillage; the doctors were insufficient to keep order; the patients who ought to have eaten fasted, those who ought to have fasted ate. From the month of June, 1854 to 1856, 41,000 men were admitted into the hospital on the Bosphorus, 4600 died whilst Miss Nightingale was at Scutari. In the first seven months the mortality was sixty per cent., which exceeded the rate of mortality in London during the cholera.

Florence Nightingale, we are told by an eye-witness, "left one bed to go to another." How she stood the mental and physical strain, is simply astounding. "The Nightingales," as she and her band of nurses were called, "have saved many lives," was written in more than one letter home; and to how many anxious hearts must the words, so simple in themselves, have brought comfort. By her influence, through her unceasing expostulation and demands, the hospital at Scutari was so cleansed, and the organisation so improved that she herself declared before the end of the war that she could conceive nothing better; and through these improved sanitary arrangements the English Army, which suffered so severely at the beginning of the campaign, was at the last almost entirely exempt from the typhus which ravaged the French Army; during the last six months the mortality was less than in England under ordinary circumstances.

But we can well imagine the days and nights of

A MESSAGE.

anxious thought she must have spent before these results were attained. The difficulties to be surmounted, the unceasing, steady patience which alone could carry the day, often against prejudice, more often still against indifference and supineness. That she did succeed is to her lasting honour, and, indifferent as she was to any personal praise or blame, still her heart must have glowed with pleasure when the following message came to her from across the sea.

It is an extract from a letter from the Queen, addressed to Mr. Sidney Herbert, and through him to Mrs. Herbert, by whom it was transmitted to Miss Nightingale.

"WINDSOR CASTLE,
"*6th December*, 1854.

"Would you tell Mrs. Herbert that I beg she would let me see frequently the accounts she receives from Miss Nightingale or Mrs. Bracebridge, as *I hear* no *details of the wounded*, though I see so many from officers, etc., about the battlefield, and naturally the former must interest *me* more than any one.

"Let Mrs. Herbert also know that I wish Miss Nightingale and the ladies would tell these poor, noble, wounded, and sick men, that *no one* takes a warmer interest or feels *more* for their sufferings, or admires their courage and heroism, *more* than their Queen. Day and night she thinks of her beloved troops. So does the Prince.

"Beg Mrs. Herbert to communicate these my words to those ladies, as I know that *our* sympathy is much valued by these noble fellows.

"VICTORIA."

Copies of this letter were made, and distributed, besides being posted up on the hospital walls and in various places. The men's gratitude knew no bounds.

One of the clergy went into most of the wards and read the letter, ending with the prayer, "God save the Queen!" to which the response was almost "startling" we are told by one present, "so hearty and vigorous from the lungs of sick and dying men came the sincere Amen."

Miss Nightingale is so inseparable from her work, that it is impossible to speak of her individually; her thoughts and feelings are to be interpreted not by words but by actions. Those long dreary corridors, many of which, when she arrived, were hardly fit for use, before Christmas time were scenes of comfort, almost of enjoyment. Groups of men gathered round the stoves, reading, or talking, or smoking; the cooking houses for men and officers were well supplied; but the comforts came from Miss Nightingale's nurses' kitchen. The Rev. J. G. Sabin, one of the most devoted army chaplains, writes:—" One meets at every turn, immense bowls of arrowroot, sago, broth, and other good things. Every man who needs such nourishment is, upon the request of the medical officers, promptly and constantly supplied. This is most valuable help to medical men, and I am always thankful that no one can now be long without the food or wine required."

And this was the work of one woman—all the gold in the Bank of England could not have accomplished such a transformation, without her head and her loving heart. Gold she needed, and it was given ungrudgingly; it was in the using of it well and wisely that she exercised her power. The love and admiration she inspired was almost marvellous.

Her own voice was seldom heard; it is through others we know her, and judge of the influence which she exercised—an influence which is still felt, perhaps even more now than when first she made use of those gifts which had come to her from God—gifts that she did not bury out of sight, but which, used for the benefit of her fellow-men, have increased exceedingly, and brought forth fruit such as even she herself could not have anticipated. Mr. Macdonald, the almoner of the *Times*, writing from the seat of the war, and from the General Hospital, just before returning to Europe, could not refrain from offering his tribute of admiration to the woman and her work, whom he had aided in every possible way himself. After tracing the growth of the hospital work, the terrible mortality, and the devotion of the medical staff, he said:—

"Wherever there is disease in its most dangerous form, and the hand of the spoiler distressingly nigh, there is that incomparable woman sure to be seen; her benignant presence is an influence for good comfort even among the struggles of expiring nature. She is 'a ministering angel,' without any exaggeration, in these hospitals, and as her slender form glides quietly along each corridor, every poor fellow's face softens with gratitude at the sight of her. When all the medical officers have retired for the night, and silence and darkness have settled down upon those miles of prostrate sick, she may be observed alone, with a little lamp in her hand, making her solitary rounds. The popular instinct was not mistaken, which, when she had set out from England on her mission of mercy, hailed her as a heroine; I trust she may not earn her title to a higher though sadder appellation. No one who has observed her fragile figure and delicate health can avoid misgivings lest these should fail. With the heart of a true woman, and the manners of a lady, accomplished and refined beyond most of her sex, she combines a surprising calmness of judgment, and promptitude and decision of character. I have hesitated to speak of her hitherto as she deserves, because I well knew that no praise of mine could do justice to her merits, while it might have tended to embarrass the frankness with which she has always accepted the aid furnished her through the Fund. As that source of supply is now nearly exhausted and my mission approaches its close, I can express myself with more freedom on this subject, and I confidently assert that but for Miss Nightingale, the people of England would scarcely, with all their solicitude, have been spared the additional pang of knowing, which they must have done sooner or later, that their soldiers even in the hospital, had found scanty refuge and relief from the unparalleled miseries with which this war has hitherto been attended."

Private letters, official documents, all alike agreed that Florence Nightingale was doing a national and a religious work, with the perfect simplicity of a true-hearted Christian woman. And yet it is almost difficult to believe, though it is alas only too true, in England, amongst her own people, there were minds sufficiently "impure and polluted," to declare that Miss Nightingale and her companions, were wanting in delicacy and refinement! "What had young women to do among wounded men?" "Why Miss Nightingale?" "Why a lady?"

A MESSAGE.

"Why not Sairey Gamp?" That awful Sairey Gamp! the thought of whom, even now, makes one's blood run cold, "reeking of onions and rum, with one hand on her patient's pillow and another in his pocket." Thank God those days are over! and it is to her, to Florence Nightingale, that we owe the change, which has made the bed of sickness and the chamber of death no longer a place of horror and fear, but a quiet haven, soothing to body and mind, healing both perhaps, or else, if the earthly temple be shattered, helping the spirit to overcome that natural fear of the unknown, and so pass in humble faith through the portals of death into life immortal. It would surely have been better for those who thus ventured to impute indelicacy to one whose stainless life bore its own testimony if they had striven to go and "do likewise." But their very meanness was a sure proof of their incapacity; they could not so much as understand the greatness of this woman, who walked so humbly and silently in the footsteps of the Christ, whose great law of love was the guiding principle of her life.

Still more difficult of belief is the fact that Miss Nightingale's opposers, not satisfied with attacking her motives, attacked her religion. They roused the "odium theologicum." She was a Papist, an Anglican, a High Church woman, a Low Church woman, a Sublapsarian, a Supralapsarian, everything and anything, except the simple Christian woman she really was.

One clergyman took occasion to warn his congregation not to send their bounty to our suffering soldiers in the East through Romish or Semi-Romish hands, when there existed safer and better channels for its conveyance. A printed letter from Mrs. Sidney Herbert was soon after circulated among his parishioners, it ran thus:—

"49 BELGRAVE SQUARE,
"9th September, 1854.

"MADAM,—By this day's post I send you a *Christian Times* of Friday week last, by which you will see how cruel and unjust are the reports you mention about Miss Nightingale and her noble work. Since then we have sent forty-seven more nurses, of which I enclose you a list. It is melancholy to think that in Christian England no one can undertake anything without these most uncharitable and sectarian attacks; and, had you not told me so, I could scarcely believe that a clergyman of the Established Church could have been the mouthpiece of such slander. Miss Nightingale is a member of the Established Church of England, and what is called rather low church; but ever since she went to Scutari, her religious opinions and character have been assailed on all points. One person writes to upbraid us for having sent her, 'understanding she is a Unitarian,' another that she is a 'Roman Catholic,' and so on. It is a cruel return to make towards one to whom all England owes so much. As to the charge of no Protestant nurses being sent, the subjoined list will convince you of its fallacy.

"We make no distinctions of creed, every one who was a good and skilful nurse was accepted, provided, of course, that we had their friends' consent, and that in other respects, as far as we could judge, they were of unexceptionable character. A large portion of the wounded being Roman Catholics, we accepted the services of some of the Sisters of Charity from St.

Stephen's Hospital in Dublin. I have now told you all, and feel sure that you will do your utmost to set these facts before those whose minds have been disquieted by these unfair and false accusations. I should have thought that the names of Mr. and Mrs. Bracebridge, who accompanied and are remaining with Miss Nightingale, would have been sufficient guarantees of the Evangelical nature of the work, but it seems nothing can stop the stream of sectarian bitterness.—I remain, Madam, Yours very faithfully,
"ELIZABETH HERBERT."

Second party of Nurses sent out the 2nd of December.

Forty-seven, viz. :—

From St. John's House	2
Protestant Ladies	10
Select Hospital Nurses, Protestant	20
Roman Catholic Sisters of Charity	15
	47

Total of first and second party, eighty-five, of whom sixty were Protestants and twenty-five Roman Catholics. The accusation, therefore, seems to fall through of itself. Nevertheless for some time there continued to appear in certain papers many acrimonious letters, which must have been intensely painful to those who loved her, and understood the singleness of heart with which she had undertaken the work, not counting the cost. What she herself felt on the subject it is difficult to ascertain. As usual she kept silence, doing her work and leaving her friends to defend her cause. Standing daily, almost hourly, face to face with suffering and death, such animosity must have seemed to her so insignificant, she had no time to dwell upon it, it could not trouble her. With 1000 sick and convalescent men to look after, closing the eyes of from thirty to forty daily in their long sleep, what thought of self could she have? Most thankfully she accepted the help of Presbyterian ministers or nurses. Her own original band of nurses was broken up and much diminished from ill health and other causes—three Sisters, three nurses, and five nuns had to be sent home ; but others came to supply the vacancies. Miss Nightingale's judgment enabled her rapidly to select the most efficient from actual observation of their work ; she looked mainly to the working powers of her band, and, with unrivalled working powers herself, soon marked who were fitting for this most difficult labour.

To those who were new to the work, and had never been subject to hospital training, the great regularity, the strict obedience to orders, must necessarily have been difficult, whereas the Catholic nuns from their habits of simple submission, possess this power remarkably.

Whilst so many were falling around her, medical men, clergymen of every denomination, this delicate, tenderly-reared woman, seemed to be endowed with a magic life, she was ever at her post, unruffled and calm, her sweet musical voice conveying the necessary orders, or speaking words of holy comfort. Her eye was everywhere, nothing was too small or insignificant for her attention, her whole soul was in her work.

At a public meeting at Exeter Hall, the Rev. J. H. Gurney in an address on "God's Heroes and the World's Heroes," when he mentioned Miss Nightingale's name, was received with cheers, which evidently came from the heart, and which were oft repeated by the immense numbers which filled the hall.

"We have lived to see a strange sight," said Mr. Gurney, "a gifted and holy woman, marked out by Providence for the blessed work of healing, dedicated to it by her own choice, summoned from her privacy by ministers of the crown who knew her worth, changing her quiet duties without a moment's hesitation for responsibilities which might have daunted one not strengthened from above, braving all that cold-hearted and narrow-minded lovers of prudery might say to her disparagement; and then assailed in print by self-styled religious men as not being perfect in her theology, as having sympathies or associations with things or persons which zealots call by a bad name, as being suspected, at anyrate, of certain right-handed or left-handed deflections, as good old Davie Deans would say, from the straight path of their orthodoxy. Truly religious partisanship has done much already to make wits merry and infidels more bold. Men of sagacious and candid minds have marvelled to see the spirit of Christianity so imperfectly reflected, so often contradicted, in the periodical literature which many serious-minded people love best. But the last exhibition is, I think, the worst, and for myself, whilst I deplore the bigotry, I wonder at the hardihood which, in the face of the English nation, could make Florence Nightingale the mark for hostile criticism, whilst the walls of Scutari resound with blessings on her name."

At another meeting, Dr. H. Kennedy, Headmaster of the Schools at Shrewsbury, pays to the "Heroine of Scutari," an equally touching tribute.

"The greater the interest and admiration with which the mission of kindness to which she had devoted herself, inspired him, the greater the delight with which he received the tidings of practical usefulness and complete success of that mission, the greater too the indignation, he would rather say the sorrow and the shame, with which he saw in the public press the vile slanders of those who strove to detract from her conduct and motives. He would not dwell upon the charge of indelicacy—a charge which could only prove the grossness of those who framed it. But she had also been called a Papist, an Anglican Papist, a Sellonite, and what not.

"Now, his own conversation with Miss Nightingale had fallen chiefly on topics of theology; and, without repeating anything said by her, he ventured to assert she was a church woman, as free from Romish sympathies as from Sectarian prejudices; that her mind dwelt in a higher and purer Christian atmosphere. Whatever her theory, she was assuredly a practical follower of Him who went about doing good; she visited the sick in their affliction, and kept herself 'unspotted from the world.'

"May God help her in this world, and reward her in the next."

If I have quoted thus at length from speeches and letters of the time, it is to show how strong was the hold which Florence Nightingale had won over the heart of the whole nation. Her honour was public property, she served the people, and high and low alike defended her, loving her for the love she gave to England's sons in the hour of their direst need.

CHAPTER VIII

"FAITHFUL UNTO DEATH."

"The air is full of farewells to the dying,
And mournings for the dead."

WHEN David was bidden choose his punishment—war, pestilence, or famine—his answer was, " I am in a great strait ; let us fall now into the hand of the Lord," and yet, surely, pestilence and famine are very terrible! War was mowing down our men; the fairest and the bravest of England's sons were laid low, and yet it was not enough!

Gradually the awful news spread that the cholera, which had played such havoc in Europe during the summer and autumn of 1854, had once more made its appearance, and this time in the midst of an army already weakened by a long winter spent in the trenches, exposed to the inclemency of an unusually severe Crimean winter. The hospitals were in as sanitary a condition as possible, the staff of medical men and the nurses in perfect working order. Nevertheless cholera of a very malignant type broke out, and made considerable ravages. Sanitary precautions hardly extended beyond the precincts of the hospitals ; if, therefore, in a temperate climate every pool or ditch be considered pregnant with disease, how much more injurious to health must these be in a country where the heat is intense, uninterrupted by cooling breezes, or unbroken by clouds and rain for weeks or months together. Fever also broke out amongst the soldiers and nurses, and could only be attributed to atmospheric influences. Of those who fell victims to this last disease was one beloved above all others, Florence Nightingale's personal friend, who had come out with her to Scutari, had seconded her from the very first, working beside her with the same self-sacrifice and renunciation which she herself displayed. Elizabeth Anne Smythe commenced her arduous work at Scutari, showing herself thoroughly fitted for its duties, so much so indeed that it was felt that her presence was desirable in a place less favoured than was the hospital over which Miss Nightingale herself ruled. She was possessed of the same powers, and had been trained by her ; when, therefore, there was such a great need for intelligent, ruling spirits, it seemed a pity to mass them in one spot. She was urged very strongly to join Miss Bracebridge at the Kululu Hospital, and after much consideration she decided to do so. Miss Nightingale was deeply grieved at losing her, and expressed her sorrow very warmly, saying, "she had hoped that they would have continued to labour together until the end of the campaign in the same hospital," but beyond these words of regret she made no effort to retain her when once she had decided that her duty lay elsewhere. And so Miss Smythe went where she thought her services were most required, beside

"FAITHFUL UNTO DEATH."

Miss Bracebridge at Kululu. She wrote a lovely letter to her friends from there, in excellent health and spirits, saying how thankful she was she had had the courage to come, and how she felt her work was even more necessary here than at Scutari, in relieving suffering and comforting the sick and wounded. Indeed, her presence was greatly appreciated, for her amiable disposition and cultivated mind rendered her society most attractive, not only to the sick but to her fellow-labourers and personal friends. A heavy shadow fell on them all when it was known that Miss Smythe was prostrate with fever. As Miss Nightingale herself said, "Martyrs there must be in every cause," and this young, beloved woman was destined to be one of the first out of that faithful band of nurses. Needless to say that all that could be done to save her life was done. For eight days medical men and nurses watched beside her, and then she gently fell asleep, to the deep sorrow of all who knew and loved her—of the soldiers she had tended, and who listened for her coming from henceforth in vain. Many a silent tear was shed when the news of her death was whispered from bed to bed, and rough men turned their faces to the wall, sorrowing for her they should never see again.

Very solemn was the funeral procession as it wended its course through the busiest streets of Smyrna to her last resting-place, in the consecrated English burying-ground. A detachment of fifty soldiers came first, then two chaplains immediately preceding the coffin, covered with a white pall emblematical of the youth and purity of her who was gone. Sisters and nurses walked on either side; both military and medical officers followed. Not a sound was heard, we are told, as they bore her that long two mile journey; multitudes had gathered along the road, standing uncovered, and a clear passage was at all times left for the procession, without having any recourse to police arrangements. And as earth was committed to earth, dust to dust, and ashes to ashes, many a tear fell, and many a sob broke forth, at the thought of the young sister they were leaving in a foreign soil, in the hope of a glorious resurrection.

The following verses were written at the time in remembrance of the gentle and much-loved nurse; a slight error was made as to the place of burial which is of little importance.

> " The streets were hushed in Scutari,
> As onward to the grave
> They bore the young and gentle nurse
> Of England's wounded brave.
>
> " The first young Christian martyr
> Is carried to the tomb,
> And busy marts and crowded streets
> Are wrapt alike in gloom.
>
> " And men who loathe the Cross and name
> Which she was proud to own,
> Yet pay their homage, meet and due,
> To her good deeds alone.
>
> " Oh, would that it were ever thus—
> That Christian deeds should shine
> With such a pure and holy light,
> To mark the source Divine;
>
> " That they who can but bless the deed
> At last may bless the name
> Of the despiséd Nazarene,
> Whom now they treat with shame.

"So, on the glorious Easter morn
  When saints and martyrs rise,
And gladly wing their angel ways
  To meet Him in the skies,

"Some happy souls, reclaimed and won
  From heathen night and gloom,
May bless the lesson taught that day
  Beside the Christian Tomb."

M. D. G.

Requiescat in pace! her work was done—she had faithfully borne her cross and now wore her crown.

Scarcely a month later Miss Nightingale left Scutari on a visit of inspection to the hospitals at Balaclava. She was received by Lord Raglan, commander in chief of the British forces, who paid her every attention, and she spent the greater part of each day in examining into the sanitary condition of the hospitals, etc. It is reported that she found them far better than she had anticipated.

Alluding to the visit, a correspondent of the *Illustrated London News* wrote as follows:—

"Among the most interesting intelligence recently received from the Crimea, are the accounts of the unwearied exertions of Miss Nightingale in the cause of suffering humanity. This excellent lady has, during her stay at Balaclava, visited the camp hospitals, and examined the arrangements in each. Throughout her inspection she was warmly greeted by the soldiers. On one of these visits Miss Nightingale went up to the hut hospitals, on the castle (or Genoese) heights, to settle three nurses, escorted by the Rev. Mr. Bracebridge, one of the chaplains, Captain Kean, R.E., Dr. Sutherland, a sergeant's guard, a boy, and eight Croats carrying baggage for the hospital. The party wound up a steep path from the harbour under the old castle, which scene is represented in the accompanying illustration."

One week afterwards the same correspondent saw this humane lady carried up to the same spot on a litter. He states, "The hospital huts, twelve in number, stand against the limestone cliffs. On the mountain side are the Marines, Rifles, and Turks; the harbour on one side, the steep cliffs where the *Prince* was lost on the other. The Genoese Castle rises on a lofty crag in front; the site is 700 feet or more above the sea, and is very airy and healthy—admirably adapted for its purpose. Here is placed Miss Nightingale's hut, beyond a small stream, the water of which is excellent, and the banks are enamelled with gay flowers. There is room for at least 800 wounded, with the best chance of recovery."

The heat during the month of May in the Crimea is very great, and exposure to the sun especially dangerous. It is supposed she must have thus exposed herself, when she went down with Mr. Sayer to the Mortar Battery, to obtain a good view of Sebastopol.* On the 15th of May, she was very unwell, and great anxiety was felt. She was staying with Mr. Bracebridge, on board the London transport in Balaclava, but she gradually grew so much worse that it was thought advisable to carry her up to the Sanitorium and place her under the immediate care of the three head physicians. The attack was a severe one, especially for a naturally delicate woman, whose constitu-

---

* The story is told that, upon the occasion of this visit, she was recognised by the 39th regiment, who sent up such a welcoming cheer as wakened up echoes in the caves of Inkerman, and startled the Russians in Sebastopol.

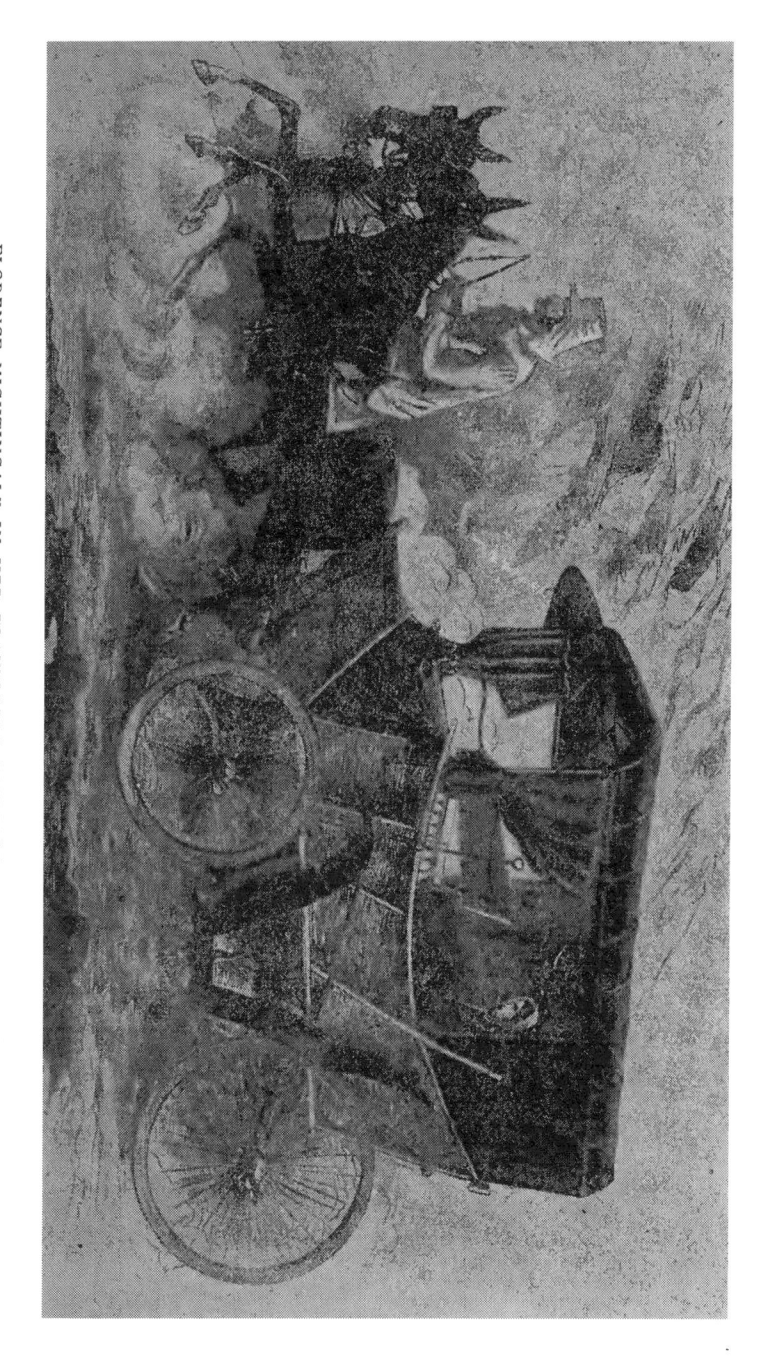

FLORENCE NIGHTINGALE IN HER TRAVELLING CARRIAGE AT THE SEAT OF WAR.

"FAITHFUL UNTO DEATH." 115

tion had been so severely tried. On more than one occasion she is said to have stood twenty hours at a stretch beside the wounded, helping the medical men. Her influence was so great, her power of persuasion so effective, that often when a patient refused to submit to an operation deemed necessary, a few words from her, her very presence beside the bed, sufficed to insure submission and quiet; but it was trying and exhausting work; so that when she was stricken by the fever great fears were entertained lest she should not have strength to resist. For several days her life was despaired of, but towards the end of the month she unexpectedly rallied, and to the great relief of those both near her and afar, anxiously awaiting news, the physicians were able to pronounce her out of danger. Her convalescence was long, but she was at last able to return to Scutari, where her presence was much needed; God had in his great mercy spared her; her work was not yet done, either in the present or in the future.

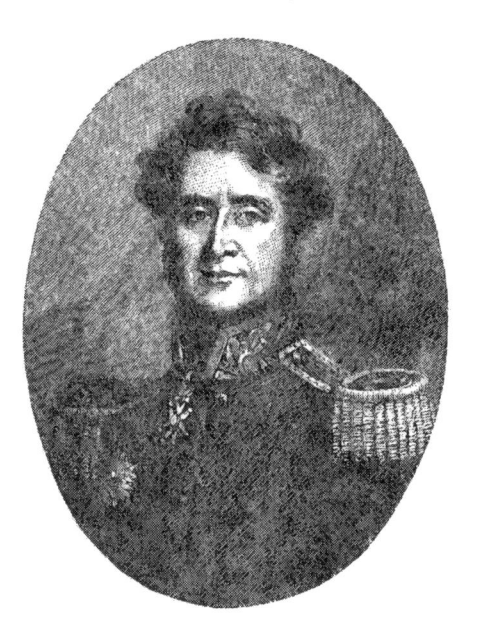

LORD RAGLAN.

She was showing the world at large what women could do, and later on she was to make that work lasting, so that her name and it should alike descend to posterity, and that many should arise and call her "blessed."

But if she escaped, others fell victims to their devotion. Three of her staff of young nurses died within a short time of each other, and were buried in the cemetery at Scutari, in the midst of the young officers and brave men they had striven to save from death. There they lie, their graves overhanging that wonderful sea of Marmora, the trees around bending to the winds, and the gold glittering mist enveloping sea and land in such marvellous brightness, that it is impossible to conceive any more perfect vision of earthly beauty; but the hearts of those who laid them to rest, even in this lovely spot, were very sad—not so much for those who were gone, as for the desolate homes, for the firesides their presence would never again brighten. Martyrs they were and are, belonging to that Holy Band who stand ever before the throne arrayed in white, with palms in their hands. Letter after letter arrived in England, telling of the comfort derived from their ministration; to quote only from one, a man writing to his mother says, "These ladies were always, from morning to night, going up and down the wards, attending to the men—sometimes washing their hands and faces, sometimes bringing them beef tea or arrowroot and such things, feeding them with their own hands, and bringing it every little while to those who were so weak that they wanted something very often. The men's rations were brought two or three times a day, and put down by the side of their couch, but often they were too weak to help themselves

"FAITHFUL UNTO DEATH."

at all. I have frequently heard a man say, 'That lady saved my life.' Miss Nightingale never waited upon me herself, but I saw her pass continually. Once I was very ill indeed, very nearly gone, and gasping for breath; there came two ladies, and stood one on each side of my couch; the lady who generally attended upon me was an elderly lady; she fetched me some weak brandy and water, and when I could

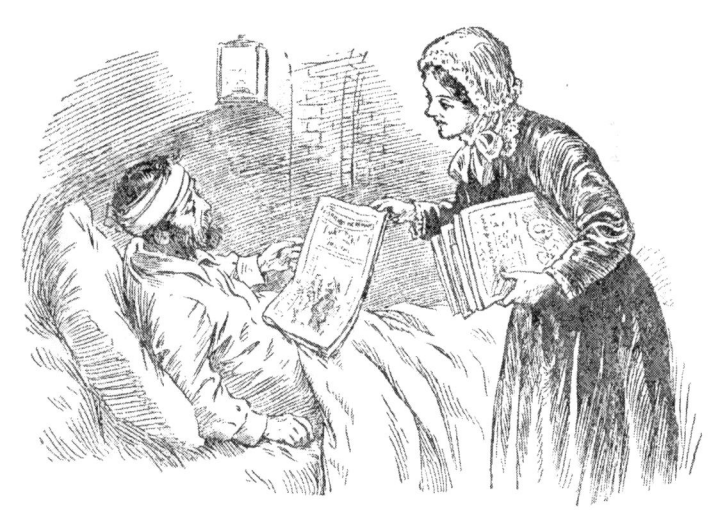

PAPERS FOR THE WOUNDED.

open my eyes I saw her leaning over me, and looking so pitiful. No one can know the good they did! Oh, I wish I could find words to say what those ladies were! Miss Nightingale always got flannels for the men, as soon as they wanted them; she took care there should always be arrowroot and such things ready for the men, when they were brought in, that they might have something directly they came."

The lack of suitable literature was greatly felt by the wounded soldiers. When this need was made known in England, Miss Nightingale's appeal was very generously responded to on all sides; many parcels of various publications were sent out, amongst these being a large quantity of the *British Workman*, which were gratefully received by the soldiers.

The early summer of 1855 seems indeed to have brought public and private sorrow to its culminating point. A year had hardly elapsed since the first cannon shots had been fired, and the three Commanders in Chiefs—the Emperor Nicholas, Marshal St. Arnaud, and, on the 28th of June, Lord Raglan—had laid down their swords and passed into another world.

On the 18th of June the terrible assault and repulse of the Redan took place, and it was to announce this defeat to the government at home that Lord Raglan penned his last dispatch. Very dark were the clouds in the horizon; Sebastopol, though attacked with unexampled bravery, still held out; " again and again," we are told, " the English renewed the assault and it was, in fact, only abandoned because there was really no one left to go on with it."

And under the shadow of this defeat Lord Raglan breathed his last. The war accounts of this time are very terrible; what sights and sounds those gentle nurses must have seen and heard, none but those who have witnessed the horrors of war can even faintly imagine. Their courage and their endurance were tested to the full, and they were not found wanting. If they fell, they fell even like their own soldiers, on the field of honour, facing the enemy!

Not till the 8th of September, did Sebastopol finally surrender to the united efforts of the allies,

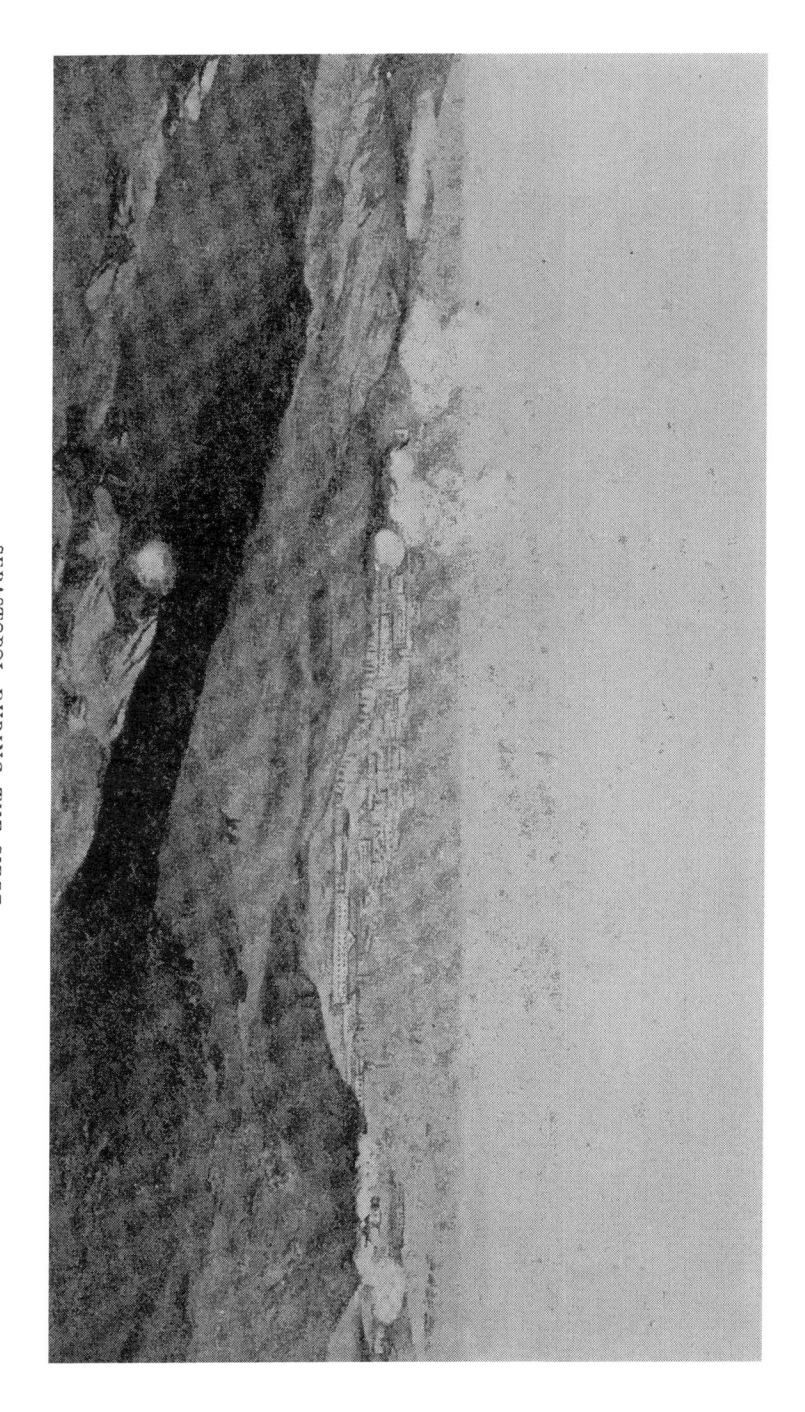

SEBASTOPOL DURING THE SIEGE.

"FAITHFUL UNTO DEATH."

and immediately there arose a cry for peace. England had tasted to the full the horrors of war. Her maimed and wounded soldiers, the "empty places" by so many firesides, testified to the severity of the struggle, and that the price of victory had been dearly paid. But now that the object had been attained, it seemed to the bulk of the nation that peace must follow immediately. Those in high places, and on the spot, knew that there was still much to be done, and that the army must needs face another Crimean winter; too much blood had been shed to allow of the conclusion of an unstable peace. Miss Nightingale and her nurses remained therefore at their posts, their services were still much needed, though the reforms they had been the means of introducing into the hospitals had borne fruit. We read in a letter from a correspondent, dated Scutari, 7th November, 1855:—"The sickness here is now far below the accommodation provided in the hospitals. The comparatively small number of invalids at present is as much owing to the superior arrangements of the hospitals, and to the high medical talent so abundantly provided, as to the sanitary condition of the camp, from which we suppose there never were fewer sick sent, since the allies first landed in the Crimea.

"The empty state of our hospitals is a pleasing contrast to that of the French.

"Two weeks ago these were fuller than they had been," etc., etc.

The example Florence Nightingale had set led others to seek consolation in the bitter sorrow which overtook them during this terrible war, by striving to help their fellow sufferers. Mrs. Willoughby Moore was the widow of the gallant soldier, Colonel Willoughby Moore, who perished in the *Europa*, refusing to leave the burning ship so long as any of his men were in it. Heart broken she looked around seeking how she could spend the remainder of her life on earth, from which all joy had departed, and nobly she bore her burden ; she organised a band of nurses and went out to Scutari to nurse and tend those very soldiers for whom her husband had laid down his life. She was nominated to the post of Lady Superintendent of the Officers' Hospital at Scutari. Her very name ensured her a welcome, and protected her from the jealousy of those in command. All through the summer and autumn she fulfilled her self-imposed duties with the greatest intelligence and devotion ; then her call came, she was laid low, and gladly she resigned her spirit into the hands of God who gave it ; how gladly, only those can know who have experienced the loneliness of earth when the best beloved has gone before and left it desolate, for truly, " Where your treasure is, there will your heart be also," and the eyes close on the sights and sounds of earth willingly, in anticipation of the joys of reunion ; but she left behind her an example to England's daughters, as her gallant husband did to England's sons. How noble it is unflinchingly to live and unflinchingly to die in the discharge of duty !

And so once more Christmas came and went, and once more the angels' song, " Peace and good will to men," ascended upwards, and with the dawn of a New Year hopes revived. Aye, surely it would be Peace, blessed peace! And in the far East the soldiers dreamed and talked of home, and of the wives and little ones awaiting their return.

CHAPTER IX.

A NATION'S GRATITUDE.

"This which thou hast done
Shall bring thee good, and bring all creatures good.
Be sure I love thee always for thy love."

G. A.

THE name of Florence Nightingale had, in the short space of one year, grown to be a household word. Everyone—even the humblest cottager whose husband, brother, or sweetheart was away at the seat of war—thought of her with tender confidence, almost feeling that the dear ones ran less danger, or, at least, that they were sure to be cared for, as long as she was there to look after and watch over them. Many were the letters she received from anxious wives and mothers, and as often as she could she sought to give comfort and strength to the forlorn.

One poor woman, the wife of a private soldier, belonging to the 39th regiment, staying with her children at South Shields, had not heard from her husband for many months; she was nearly heartbroken, and reduced to great straits, suddenly the idea came to her to write to Miss Nightingale. She did so, and a few weeks later received the following letter, which shows well the tender sympathy of the woman who wrote it :—

"SCUTARI BARRACK HOSPITAL,
"5th March.

"DEAR MRS. LAWRENCE, — I was exceedingly grieved to receive your letter, because I have only sad news to give you in return. Alas! in the terrible time we had here last year, when we lost from seventy to eighty men per day in these hospitals alone, many widows have had to suffer like you, and your husband was, I regret to say, amongst the number. He died in this hospital, 20th February, 1855, just at the time when our mortality reached its height, of fever and dysentery, and on that day we buried eighty men.

"In order that I might be sure that there was no mistake of name, and that there were not two men of the same name, I wrote up to the colonel of his regiment, who confirms the sad news in the note I enclose; and though he is mistaken in the precise date of your husband's death, there is no mistake, alas! in the fact.

"I wished to get this reply before I wrote to you. Your husband's balance, due to you, was £1, 2s. 4½d., which was remitted home to the Secretary of War, 25th September, 1855, from whom you can have it on application.

"As you were not aware of being a widow, you are, of course, not in receipt of any allowance as a widow; you should therefore make application to Lieutenant Colonel Lefroy, R.A., Honorary Secretary

Patriotic Fund, 16a Great George Street, Westminster, London.

"I enclose the necessary papers for you to fill up. Your Colonel's letter will be sufficient proof of your husband's death. I enclose it for that purpose. You will state all particulars about your children.

"Your minister will help you to fill it up.

"I am very sorry for you and your trouble. Should you have any difficulty about the Patriotic Fund, you must make use of this letter, which will be sufficient evidence for you to produce of your being a widow.

"With sincere sympathy for your great loss, I remain, yours truly, FLORENCE NIGHTINGALE."

I have given the letter without curtailing it, because it shows so thoroughly the character of her who wrote it. Nothing that can help the sorrow-stricken widow to bear her burden is omitted; little details, so necessary, are dwelt upon with great common sense, in which there is no touch of harshness, only pity and a desire to afford help; there are the children to be thought of, material needs, the necessity for personal exertion hinted at, so as to rouse the mourner, and all so delicately done, to give as little pain as possible. No wonder those who came into daily contact with her loved her well!

At last the much longed for peace dawned over Europe, and with the early spring, with the flowers and the songs of birds, hope revived in many hearts; and if some were sad, longing with that imperious yearning which no earthly power can overcome—

> "For the touch of a vanished hand,
> And the sound of a voice that is still,"

the cry was smothered, and the aching heart bowed

low on "Thanksgiving day," striving for submission to the will of the All Father. Alas! the spirit is oft times willing, but the flesh is weak.

To the very last Florence Nightingale remained at her post, and then, fearful of the ovation which she knew would be hers if she attempted to return to England publicly, under her own name, she travelled quietly from the East with her aunt, under the name of Mrs. and Miss Smith. Her fellow-passengers little guessed who the quiet, graceful woman was, travelling home! The incognito served her well; after nearly two years' absence she returned to her father's house as quietly as she had left it. But she could not long remain thus hidden; congratulations poured in from every side. The workmen of a large manufactory in the neighbourhood of Newcastle-on-Tyne sent a most touching address, congratulating her on her safe return to her home and friends, to which she replied :—

"*23rd August*, 1856.

"MY DEAR FRIENDS,—I wish it were in my power to tell you what was in my heart when I received your letter.

"Your welcome home, your sympathy with what has been passing while I have been absent, have touched me more than I can tell in words. My dear friends, the things that are the deepest in our hearts are perhaps what it is most difficult for us to express.

"'She hath done what she could.' These words I inscribed on the tomb of one of my best helpers when I left Scutari. It has been my endeavour, in the sight of God, to do as she has done.

"I will not speak of reward when permitted to do

our country's work—it is what we live for—but I may say to receive sympathy from affectionate hearts like yours is the greatest support, the greatest gratification that it is possible for me to receive from man.

"I thank you all, the 1800, with grateful, tender affection. And I should have written before to do so, were not the business, which my return home has not ended, almost more than I can manage.—Pray, believe me, My dear friends, Yours faithfully and gratefully, FLORENCE NIGHTINGALE."

It is scarcely to be wondered at if the whole nation, from the Queen to the humblest of her subjects, was desirous of publicly testifying the deep gratitude, the respect and love, which was the universal feeling towards her.

Of wealth she had enough and to spare; materially, she needed nothing, even from the praise of men she shrank sensitively; for love of her fellows she had laboured to help poor humanity—Christ-like, she had not counted the cost—she had given freely, asking nothing in return. And now she had come home once more to her father's house, to recover that health and strength which she had expended in the service of her country. Whilst England was busy with her name, whilst every heart was overflowing with gratitude, she was wandering once more in the old haunts of her childhood, with sister, father, mother, and devoted friends, all thankful that God had vouchsafed to spare her life in the midst of the many and great dangers through which she had passed.

It was the Prince Consort himself who suggested the design of the jewel which Her Majesty Queen Victoria presented to Miss Nightingale.

All the purest imaginings of poetry, religion, and art were expressed in this royal gift from the Queen of England to her who had faced death in the fulfilment of a self-imposed duty for God and for her country, and who above all other women, she, the lady of the land, must, therefore, "delight to honour."

A St. George's cross in ruby-red enamel, on a white field representing England. This is encircled by a black band, typifying the office of charity, on which is inscribed a golden legend, "Blessed are the merciful." The royal donor is expressed by the letters V.R. surmounted by a crown in diamonds impressed upon the centre of the St. George's cross, from which also rays of gold emanating upon the field of white enamel are supposed to represent the glory of England. Wide-spreading branches of palm, in bright green enamel, tipped with gold, form a framework for the shield, their stems at the bottom being banded with a ribbon of blue enamel (the colour of the ribbon for the Crimean medal), on which in golden letters is inscribed "Crimea." At the top of the shield, between the palm branches, and connecting the whole, three brilliant stars of diamonds illustrate the idea of the light of heaven shed upon the labours of mercy, peace, and charity, in connection with the glory of a nation. On the back of this royal jewel is an inscription on a golden tablet, written by Queen Victoria, recording it to be a gift and testimonial in memory of services rendered to her brave army by Miss Nightingale.

The jewel is about three inches in depth, by two and a-half in width. It is to be worn, not as a brooch or ornament, but rather as the badge of an order.

A NATION'S GRATITUDE.

This gift was accompanied by an autograph letter full of deep feeling and graceful, queenly kindness.

Long before Miss Nightingale left her post and returned home, the nation was busy with the thought of how it could acknowledge, in a manner acceptable to her, the heroic work she had accomplished.

It was well that all should understand the work which had been done—the radical change her personal heroism and the courage with which she had dared public opinion, had brought about in the position of woman. She had opened out a new sphere of action for the many unemployed, whose lives were frittered away in that most terrible of all lots—inaction.

Those who were best acquainted with Florence Nightingale knew, that to enable her to continue the work she had begun, to make use of that wonderful power of organisation and command which genius alone possesses, would be to her the most acceptable proof of their appreciation. At a grand monster meeting at Manchester, convened to decide what form the testimonial should take, the Hon. Mr. Sidney Herbert, after dwelling upon her achievements, said : " Her self-devotion has been truly great, but it has not been greater than that of the other ladies who accompanied her; and, mind you, when we talk of a testimonial to Miss Nightingale, it is to the honour, not of Miss Nightingale only, but to the honour of all those ladies, all those persons of whatever class who have accompanied her and rendered her assistance. She is distinguished above all others by the influence she can exercise over others, and by the extraordinary powers of organisation and administration which she has displayed. These are the peculiarities of Miss

Nightingale, which point her out as the person to whom this great reform of our hospital system ought to be entrusted.

"But some have objected. If she has done so much, why saddle her with more? They do not know Miss Nightingale who utter that opinion. She is one to whom, 'life is real, life is earnest.' She looks for her reward in this country in having a fresh field for her labours, and the means of extending the good she has already begun. Depend upon it, you cannot pay her a compliment dearer to her heart than in giving her more work to do. She wants the means to continue the work she has begun, and I look upon this meeting as most important, because I know the position Manchester occupies in England—and I know how much this meeting may do to set an example which will spread, and I trust that the testimonial to Miss Nightingale will be one to make her influence felt all over England, and at the same time be worthy of the occasion which has called it forth—worthy of the lady in whose honour we have met, and worthy, I must also say, of the gratitude of a great nation, to whom she has rendered immortal services."

Other voices were raised in public and in private to impress the same idea upon all minds—not for herself, but for her work. To break through the old routine and establish a new order of things, and having established it, to make it a permanent institution. From North to South of England the words were repeated, meetings upon meetings followed each other; with regard to the subscriptions, a resolution was passed embodying the prevailing sentiment that they should be as general as possible, in order to show the universal appreciation of Miss Nightingale's labours, but that large individual subscriptions were both uncalled for and undesirable. The chief thing was, that the debt of the nation should be paid; it mattered little to the mass what form the tribute of love and gratitude should take, so long as the world should see that England knew how to honour one who "in the eyes of the world had done honour to her." But on one point all were agreed, that she was to be allowed perfect freedom of action, to do what she thought best, unhampered by sectarianism or the will of others; she had proved herself worthy of the faith and trust of all men, having but one earnest desire to accomplish the will of Him who said, "Come ye blessed, . . . for I was an hungered, and ye gave Me meat; I was thirsty, and ye gave Me drink; . . . naked and ye clothed Me; I was sick, and ye visited Me!"

And thus it came to pass that the English people, rich and poor alike, the widow and the orphan, whose husband and father she had tended, dropped their mite into the common purse and placed in her loyal hands the nation's offering —its thank-offering—for the good which she, a tender woman, had done; for the love she had poured out so ungrudgingly. Fifty thousand pounds they gave her, to found a home which should for ever bear her name, and where other women should learn to tend the sick, wisely and well as she had done, in the same spirit of love and self-sacrifice, remembering the words of their Lord and Master, "Inasmuch as ye have done it unto one of the least of these My brethren, ye have done it unto Me."

CHAPTER X.

ADIEU.

"There is a tear for all who die,
　　A mourner o'er the humblest grave;
But nations swell the funeral cry—
　　And triumph weeps above the brave.

"For them is sorrow's purest sigh
　　O'er ocean's heaving bosom sent;
In vain their bones unburied lie—
　　All earth becomes their monument."

THUS it came to pass that, before the close of 1856, one of the greatest battle-fields of Europe was deserted, and where the roar of the cannon had resounded for so long where so many noble hearts had ceased to beat, silence and peace reigned.

Before Florence Nightingale left the scene of her labours she marked the spot by an everlasting sign—on the heights of Balaclava, where English courage and heroism had shone so brightly before the whole of Europe, she caused a gigantic cross to be raised, upon which was inscribed, "Lord, have mercy upon us."

ADIEU.

This was her final adieu to the land where, for two years, she had laboured. To the Divine mercy she committed the results of her work—the souls alike of the living and the dead, whom He had delivered into her hand.

The sailors, as they sail by, can see it towering upwards to the sky, bringing to their remembrance a woman's love and a woman's work. Along the shores of the Black Sea, in the wasted plains of the Crimea, save for the ruins which time alone could repair, with the evacuation of the troops, life resumed its everyday aspect. Both French and English were anxious to be gone, and their departure was rapidly effected; towards the end of the summer and early autumn of that year, 1856, all that remained to bear testimony to the struggle which had been waged so fiercely, was the rows of graves, with their monumental crosses and slabs, in the burial ground, on the low cliffs of the Sea of Marmora. As the soldiers stood on the decks of the great ships, which were bearing them home to their loved ones, many of them must have raised their eyes and gazed sadly on those graves of lost comrades, glittering in the sun.

It is a lovely spot, hanging above the blue waters, mid-way, as it were, between earth and heaven. A sacred spot to all English hearts must this burial-ground of Scutari ever be, from generation to generation. To the spot where our heroes lie awaiting the great resurrection, a grateful nation will ever turn in reverential awe. Many a traveller will wander between those rows of graves reading the names, the dates, roughly hewn sometimes, with a sense of pity as if they had been lain there but yesterday. The dead are always young, they never age; as they looked when we bade them the last farewell, so they will ever remain in our memories. Time passes over them, it cannot touch so much as a stray curl on the head we loved so well, but it is better to lift our eyes from earth to heaven, and to strive to think of them, not as they were, but as they are, in the "many mansions."

A lesson is taught us by the memorial which Queen Victoria and her people raised to the memory of the heroes who fell in the Crimean War. No broken column is there, no pagan insinuation that life was ended. A Christian in heart and soul was he who designed that memorial, worthy of England, worthy of our Queen. We sorrow not as those without hope. Life was but dawning for those whose mortal bodies lie within the sound of the surging waves!—the testimony is there for those who will understand.

"A square marble base, surmounted by four figures of angels with drooping wings, supporting between them a tapering shaft which *rises towards the sky.*"

There it stands, telling us of those young lives, not lost but gone before; lifting our souls upwards, ever upwards, with strange yearning; away from earth and its battlefields through that "portal we call Death," into the "Life elysian."

Such is the Christian hope; and there we have laid our dead, in the glorious sunshine—very different from the Turkish cemetery which lies a cannon shot more inland. Its dark and celebrated cypress trees, in thousands upon thousands, form a picturesque background to the landscape.

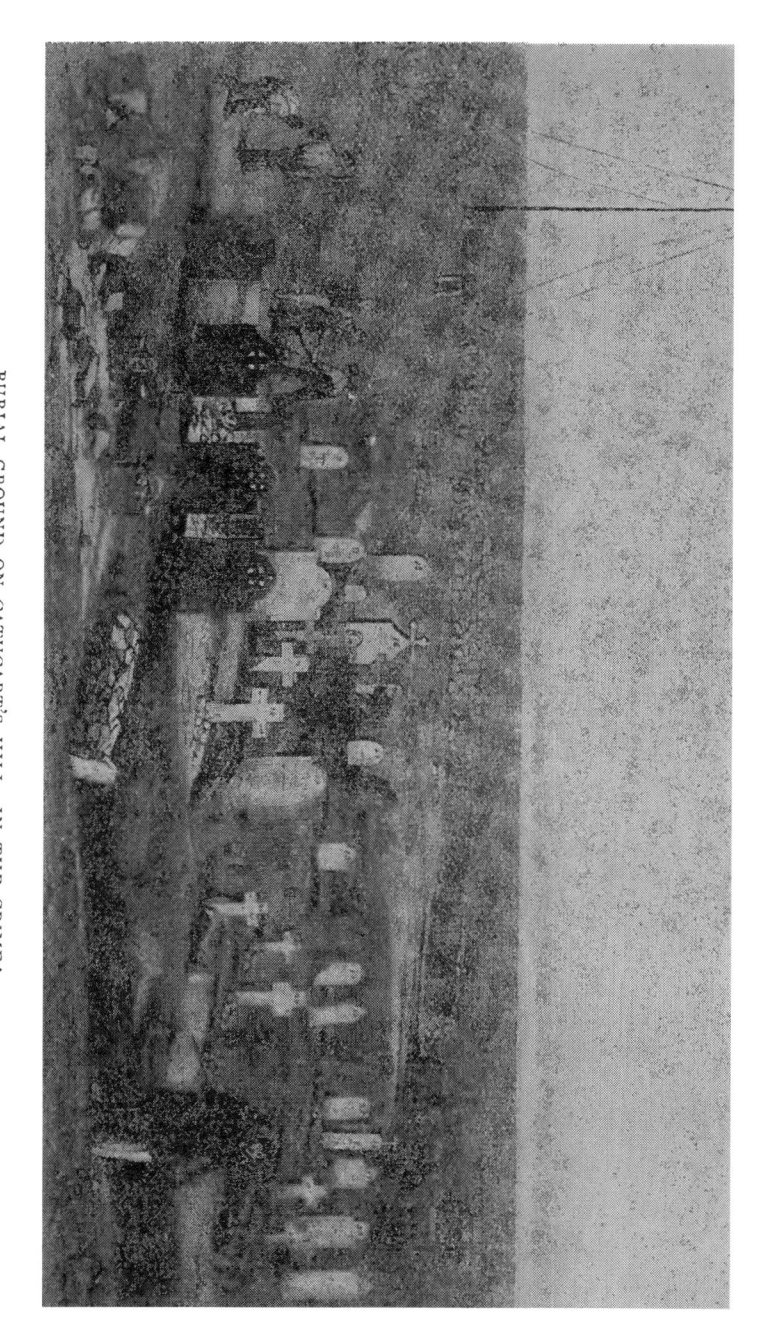

BURIAL GROUND ON CATHCART'S HILL, IN THE CRIMEA.

The smiling eastern sky, the glorious sunlight, the silvery rays of the moon, are all alike powerless to dispel the deep solemn gloom of that mass of cypress trees. Walking in their shadow one feels as if life and light were alike unknown. The joyous songs of the birds, the merry hum of the insects, the echo of the sea, all seem swallowed up in death ; the effect is awful and startling.

Of this cemetery there is a strange legend told, weird and awful in its significance, but which may interest our readers. It forms a speaking contrast to our faith, and the quiet resting-place of our dead ; it is told as follows :—

" Myriads of birds about the size of a thrush frequent the dark shades, hover over the tombs, and flit noiselessly from that sea of storms, the Euxine, to the fairer Sea of Marmora, where they turn and retrace their flight, often touching the masts of the vessels that sail beneath them.

" They have never been seen to stop or feed, and they have never been heard to sing ; all their life seems passed in flitting from one sea to another. No one has as yet discovered exactly what kind of birds these phantom wanderers are, for it is asserted that a dead one has never been seen, and the Moslems hold them in such veneration that they will not permit one to be killed.

"All that is known of them is that they have a dark plumage, and blue feathers on the breast.

" During the tempestuous weather which so frequently disturbs the waves of the Bosphorus, when these birds can no longer flit in mid-air, they desert the sea for the land and take shelter in the cypress groves. At these times, when the storm rages and

Boreas himself seems unchained, and to be pouring destruction on the many vessels that crowd the surrounding waters, the birds emit a loud sound—not a melodious sound, or a soft warble, but a shrill sharp cry as of agony. This thrilling sound has caused the Turks to declare that they are the condemned souls, who, having lived an evil life in this world, are not permitted to rest quiet in the tomb by the side of their holier brethren; and as the Turk loves quiet, no greater penance could be laid upon his spirit."

Such is the Mohammedan legend, and in the darkness of those cypress trees, with no whispered hope of a bright hereafter, their dead lie.

How often the thoughts of those who sailed homewards must have hovered over the Christian burial-ground, where the comrade and friend slept his last sleep; how many a memento, a flower, a stone, was carried home to the mourners, and cherished tenderly, wept over with many a tear of mingled grief and pride. But joy was nevertheless the paramount feeling. France and England rejoiced, welcoming home their heroes, each country vying with the other to do honour to their soldiers. On the breast of many a Frenchman the Victoria Cross was proudly worn, and French decorations were equally distributed in the English army.

But no sight could have been more touching than when Queen Victoria distributed the medals to those to whom they had been awarded. With her intuitive delicacy our late beloved Queen understood that it was for her and for England they had suffered; from her hand, therefore, it was meet their reward should come, and so, with her two young sons beside her, she stood to receive her heroes. " Gaunt, pallid forms,

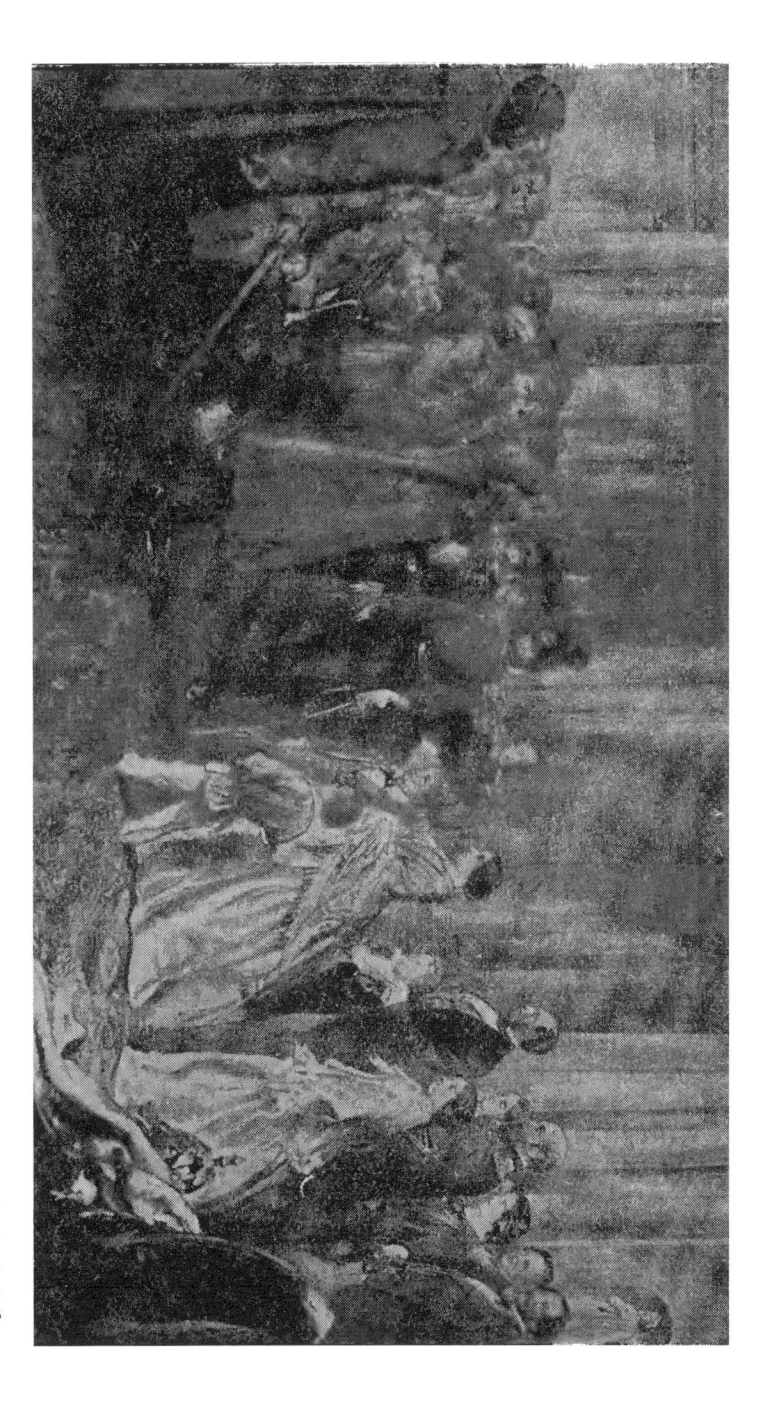

From a Painting] QUEEN VICTORIA PRESENTING MEDALS TO THE CRIMEAN VETERANS. [*by Sir J. Gilbert.*

mutilated and maimed, hobbling along on crutches, or staggering along on sticks. For officers and men alike the Queen had a kindly word of sympathy which drew tears from many eyes, and, occasionally singling out a private soldier who bore upon his breast more than the usual number of decorations, raising by some well-deserved and well-timed compliment the blush of modest and humble merit upon his manly cheek."

The Queen exerted herself to be the first to welcome her brave army home. We read in a paper of the time :—

"The Queen shot over rapidly to Portsmouth to meet the 8th Hussars, who had just arrived from the Crimea. The Hussars passed by Her Majesty in slow time, and were followed by one hundred and fifty of the invalids walking, four omnibuses were full of those who could not walk and the litters of those going to the hospital."

There were reviews and peace celebrations all over the land. At the Crystal Palace the "Scutari Monument" by Baron Marochetti, and the "Peace Trophy" were unveiled in the presence of the Queen, surrounded by a guard of soldiers who had served in the Crimea, each wearing his medal!

The "Peace Trophy" represented a "large allegorical figure of Peace, clad in silver and gold, with a real olive branch in the right hand."

Peace! peace! resounded throughout the land, from the palace to the cottage. Not a village but welcomed back its hero, not one of whom but spoke in hushed voices reverentially of the "ladies" who had nursed and tended them. "But for the nurses I should have died," more than one said.

No marvel then if the "Nightingale Fund" prospered. The £50,000 presented to Miss Nightingale, to enable her to found a Training School for nurses, was the out-pouring of a nation's gratitude. It was especially stipulated that no large donations were desired, the widow's and the orphan's mite were most welcome. Love was to be the foundation stone upon which the new system was to be built up. Love entails self-sacrifice, but it is not visible, it is hardly even felt. The joy of giving, the power of self-renunciation, are the offspring of true love, and the flowers and fruit they bear are so delicate of texture, so beautiful, a very "joy for ever," to the giver and to the receiver.

"A Home," from whence all that was pure and good should emanate; from whence women should go forth, carrying with them the lamp of knowledge and power, as well as love, to lighten the dark places of the earth, even as she their founder had carried her lamp through the dark wards of the Scutari Hospital.

Such was the purpose of the "Nightingale Home."

CHAPTER XI.

IN MEMORIAM.

"The real dignity of a gentlewoman is a very high and unassailable thing, which silently encompasses her from her birth to her grave."—*Miss Nightingale.*

FROM the time of her return to England, after the Crimean campaign, Miss Nightingale's active life may be considered ended. From henceforth she was a confirmed invalid, often for weeks together confined to her room. But if the flesh was weak the spirit was still willing, heart and brain were alike active in continuing the work she had begun. From her couch she organised, made plans, and answered the numerous letters which were continually being addressed to her. It is impossible to conceive the extent of her correspondence and her literary work. At home and abroad her advice was sought; quoting her own words she had hardly "ten minutes of idle time in the day."

It is well that the daughters of England should recognise the fact that if "England expects every man to do his duty," the same rule applies to the women of England. Florence Nightingale opened out the path, treading under her feet idle prejudices, not flaunting the vexed question of woman's rights, but ably proving that there is work which no man's hand can do, that in love and tender pity our power lies, that the sceptre we wield needs no legislation to maintain its supremacy—it is upheld by the great law of Nature and Nature's God. Love! therein lies our greatest power, that which has ruled the world ever since its creation, for weal or woe. And the lesson which Florence Nightingale has striven to teach the women of the nineteenth century is this, that work and love united is an irresistible lever, making strong the weakest, overcoming difficulties, an arbiter between life and death; and both by precept and example she has shown her fellow-countrywomen what is requisite to enable them rightly to use this power.

Firstly, by knowledge. She has written much and wisely on all that concerns health and sanitary arrangements in England and abroad. In her "Notes on Nursing," for the labouring classes, the most simple rules are laid down, such as can help the ignorant to alleviate suffering. and make the sick room a place of healing, not of death as alas it is too often, from want of knowledge.

Her great literary work, the one upon which she expended the most time, thought, and care, is "Notes on Matters affecting the Health, Efficiency, and Hospital Administration of the British Army." She was able in this work to speak with authority, what she brought to bear on the subject being founded chiefly on her own experience of the wars. "Notes on Hospitals," published in 1863, was also written with perfect knowledge of her subject, owing in a great measure to her foreign travels which enabled her to appreciate the good and bad points in their construction. The block system evidently met with her approbation. Her attention was next drawn to India, to its sanitary condition, and the possibility of life there.

"Life and Death in India," from her pen, was a paper read at the National Association for Promotion of Social Science at Norwich in 1873.

Every now and again, as long as her strength would permit, she spoke to those labourers who were working in the field she herself had opened out to them, encouraging their efforts, bidding them persevere in that life of self-sacrifice upon which they had entered. Reading what she has written, one feels how thoroughly she understood those she was addressing, that their trials had been her trials, their disappointments her disappointments; and this evidence of sympathetic knowledge adds ten times to the value of her teaching, for, even as Chaucer describes the "poure Persoun of a town,"

"This noble ensample to his sheep he gaf,
That first he wroughte and afterward he taughte."

Those who have never worked cannot understand the labourer, those who have never suffered, the sufferer; but the memory of all these things may fail, papers may be lost, the ink may grow pale and illegible, even as the hand which traced the words will lie powerless in the grave, but England and the English people decreed that Florence Nightingale's work should not die, that, on the contrary, it should go on increasing and bearing fruit. Therefore it was that a wing in St. Thomas' Hospital was devoted

K

to the training of nurses for hospital work. The fifty thousand pounds subscribed by the nation were devoted to this purpose—the founding of the "Nightingale Home."

Very curious is the history of the site upon which St. Thomas' Hospital now stands. We know well those blocks of buildings on the Surrey side of Westminster Bridge, and, strange to say, from time immemorial that spot seems to have been chosen as best suited for works of charity. In ransacking old papers we have found it recorded that, soon after the conquest, a convent was erected on the very spot where the "Home" now stands.

The donor was a pious woman named Mary, who had acquired a large fortune by the heritage of a boat to convey passengers across the Thames, there being at that time no bridge over the river. For this reason the woman bore the Saxon appellation of "over—rie" —*i.e.*, "over the river." For about two hundred years the convent flourished and doubtless did much good, but in 1212 it was destroyed by fire. In the year 1213 we find an Almoney had been erected on the spot for indigent children and necessitous proselytes; how long this continued to exist we do not exactly know; the next change was made by a Bishop of Winchester, who took a small "edifice" there because of "the salubrity of the air and the purity of the water." It was surrounded by high trees, and the meadows were "sweet and abundant." Here the good bishop founded a hospital; there was a master and brethren, also sisters to attend and nurse the poor. Probably this state of things continued until the Reformation, when old things were done away with and a new order was instituted. Still there is a feeling that this spot, once so fair with sweet meadows and tall waving trees beside the river side, now so busy, as the centre of a great city with an ever-increasing population, was as it were consecrated to works of charity. When old St. Thomas' was pulled down, the block system, so highly appreciated by Miss Nightingale, was adopted for the new buildings, and it was one of these blocks that was appropriated by the "Nightingale Home."

The Home was originally opened in Surrey Gardens under the superintendence of Mrs. Wardroper. Miss Crossland was then the Superintendent, and was at the head of the "Home" for seventeen years. A conversation with this lady is still very vivid in my mind, showing, as it did, how deep her interest was in the work, and how entirely she was imbued with the same feelings, the same principle of action as Miss Nightingale herself.

The "Home" is thus described: "A large entrance Hall bright with flowers greets the visitor; over the door leading into the nurses' sitting-room are the words—

"'Love suffereth long and is kind.

"'Love envieth not itself, is not puffed up.

"'Doth not behave unseemly.

"'Seeketh not her own, is not easily provoked.

"'Thinketh no evil.'

"A clock, the gift of the grand Duchess of Baden, and a bust of Sir Harry Verner, President of the Council, occupy one panel. Further on is a marble bust of Miss Nightingale, but the greatest attraction is a full length marble figure of her, carefully protected by a glass case, representing her in her Crimean nurses' dress, carrying in her hand the lamp with which it was her wont to glide from bed to bed along the hospital wards, to see that the Doctor's orders were carried out, and that there was no especial case requiring immediate attention. 'The lady with the lamp,'—under that title she will go down to posterity. In the centre of the wall as one enters, facing the inscription we have already given, is one of her Christmas gifts to the Home, a motto in illuminated letters:—

"'To hands that work and eyes that see,
Give wisdom's heavenly lore,
That whole and sick, and weak and strong
May praise Thee evermore.'

"A small, simply furnished room leading out of the hall is the Superintendent's private room. There are thirty-four probationers, who are distributed amongst the different wards, attend lectures, and are instructed in everything necessary to make them thoroughly efficient nurses. Thirty-eight was the number which formed the first band that accompanied Miss Nightingale to the Crimea; mentioning the fact I was assured that it was quite unintentional, a mere chance, if there is such a thing in this world as chance!

"Each nurse has her own private room. A Chapel is attached to the home; over the Communion table is a picture by Horsley of the 'Raising of Jairus's daughter.'"

And so it comes to pass, that year after year women go forth out of this "Home," well taught, loving their work, not feeling it a hardship, smiling at the idea of self-sacrifice. They have their reward in the many cases of healing, which, thanks to their wise care, restore wives to their husbands, and save many a

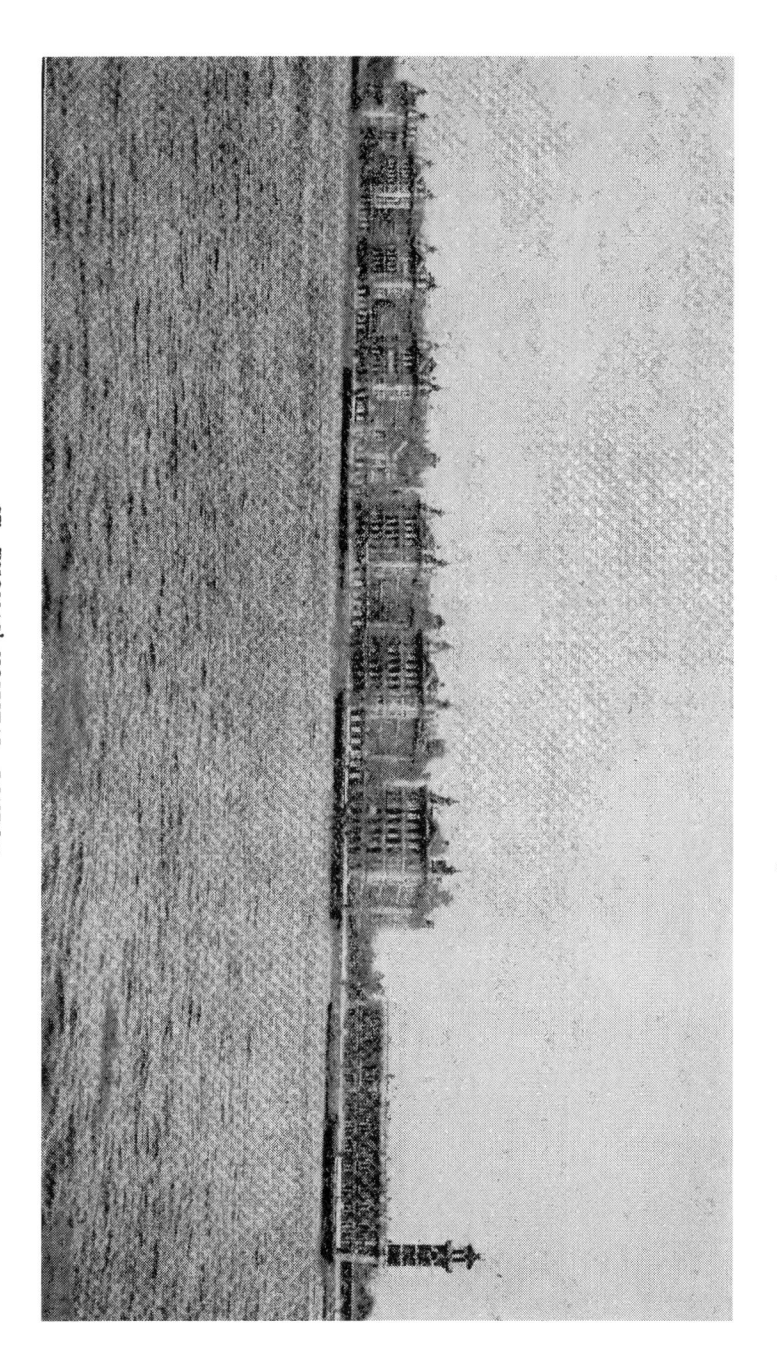

ST. THOMAS' HOSPITAL, LONDON.

NIGHTINGALE HOME.
*

home from the dark shadow of widowhood and orphanage; and for the workers themselves, empty lives have been made full; instead of days frittered away in idleness and discontent, the noblest joy is theirs—helping others to bear life's burdens. From her retirement Miss Nightingale looked forth upon a world which she helped to make more tender, more Christ-like.

And so, as the shadows of evening gathered around her, and the light of her earthly lamp paled, heavenly light but shone the brighter. Yet there were many long years of quiet waiting, of bodily if not mental inaction, and of absolute seclusion from the world, ere the eternal gates were thrown open, and her Master's voice spoke the glorious words: "Well done, thou good and faithful servant. Enter thou into the joy of thy Lord."

CHAPTER XII.

HOME AT LAST.

FLORENCE NIGHTINGALE had never been physically strong, and the tremendous strain of those terrible months in the Crimea left her permanently bankrupt as to health. Although her life was prolonged far beyond anything her friends could have dared to hope, and even outstripped the normally allotted span, she was always more or less of a confirmed invalid. This fact assisted her in preserving that complete retirement which her modest nature craved, and excused her from the, to her, trying ordeal of appearing as an object of public admiration. But it was impossible that she should be forgotten. The halo which surrounded her name was a light that could not be hidden. And although, if the newspapers busied themselves about her whether she would or no, and reporters being forbidden to penetrate the sanctuary of her private life, no published details of her doings could be regarded as authentic, yet every child in the land became familiar with the picture of the sweet-faced woman with the lamp, giving drink to a wounded soldier in the night watches, and it was as though of her also had the Divine words been spoken, "Wheresoever this"—the story of the Crimea—should be told "in the whole world, there shall also this, that this woman hath done, be told for a memorial of her."

Nevertheless, those long, long years of seclusion were not idle. As we have already said her advice and encouragement were always ready for those who needed them, and by means of letters to national societies on social subjects she continued to disseminate in writing the principles on which she had worked, and from which she had herself reaped such good results; while the almost mysterious silence with which she surrounded her comings and goings, only served to heighten the impressiveness and increase the preciousness of the words she sent forth. When she spoke, it was as if in a voice that reached us from another world, and all listened with reverence.

Florence Nightingale was one of those rare examples of women whom all people, rich and poor, high and low, delight to honour. No mark of esteem which the King or nation could bestow was lacking to her: the Red Cross from Queen Victoria; the dignity of Lady of Grace of the Order of St. John of Jerusalem by King Edward; in November, 1907, the Order of Merit was bestowed upon her, she being the only woman upon whom that exceptional distinction was conferred; the Lord Mayor, as we have already said, offered her the greatest distinction in his power, and on her last birthday, the day she attained her ninetieth year, King Edward the Seventh sent her his congratulations, while friends and admirers of lesser rank almost overwhelmed her with gifts of flowers. Surely these last tributes must have made her heart glad—she who was born in the land of flowers!

Just three months later, on the 13th of August,

1910, Florence Nightingale closed her eyes on the things of this world and fell asleep, to wake in that other world, for which her soul must have longed in those last years of her earthly pilgrimage.

He came suddenly at the last, that angel of death, with healing on his wings, and a strange thrill ran through the heart of the whole nation when the news spread abroad, and was whispered from one to the other, "Florence Nightingale is dead!" It was but a short time before that the words, "The King is dead," had struck a similar note of sorrow and consternation. Both of them had been workers, not for themselves but for others, for the country and the people they loved. The one died in harness, the other lay long in her virginal whiteness, waiting for the angel's call.

So, crowned with age and honour, she passed away from this world, but not from the hearts of her countrymen. There she will reign supreme; she will have no rival, save perhaps the great Queen who loved and honoured her, and who looked to her in those dark Crimean days for news of "our dear soldiers."

We have told how silence surrounded her during the last years of her life; but when the doors of her earthly home were thrown open, and she was carried forth, that silence was broken; there was a murmuring of many voices, telling of the good deeds she had done, and those acts of loving kindness which have made of her name a household word.

That her mortal remains should lie in Westminster Abbey beside the great men and women of her country—poets, statesmen, warriors, philanthropists —was the natural desire of the nation, but it was not

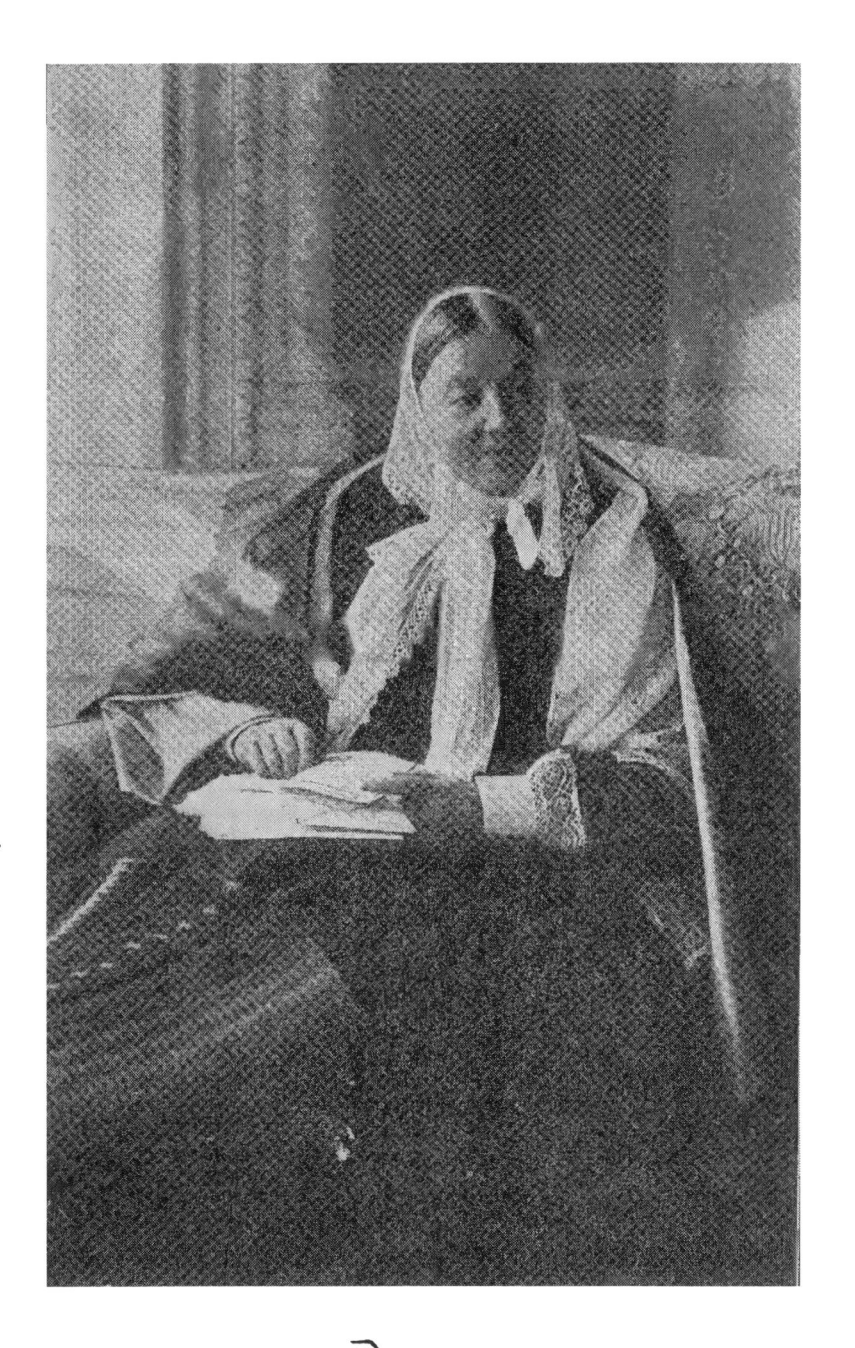

Florence Nightingale

hers. She did not see herself as others saw her—of herself she had done nothing; it was God who had inspired her, she was but a tool in His hands, and she gave God the glory.

She knew the heart of the people, how they loved her, how they would claim her, that she should lie forever and forever in their midst; but she yearned after her own people, and the home of her childhood. To lie beside her father and mother, away from the busy world, in the open country, that was what she desired. And so strongly and earnestly did she make this desire known, that there was no putting it on one side; indeed, from the first there was no thought of doing so, her will had been law with the many during her life, it would be sacred after her death, and so without a murmur London let her go.

Tears, not of sorrow but of grateful joy, were shed as she passed through the streets of the metropolis for the last time, flowers, which she loved so dearly, covering the mortal remains of her who had given her life, her strength, and her intellect for her fellow-creatures. Almost unbeknown she went on her way, a nation's heroine. Eight stalwart soldiers awaited her at each stage of this her last journey. On their shoulders they bore the white-draped coffin with its load of flowers, from hearse to station, on her journey home.

Through the abbey town of Romsey they bore her, along roads familiar to her childhood; past her home, Embley Park, ever on and on, until at last they reached the old church of East Willow there, and her faithful guardsmen carried her through a crowd of simple country folk who had known and loved her, into the church where she had been wont to pray.

The outside world had nothing more to do with her; God claimed her for His own, and mother earth received into her bosom the fragile casket of one who had spent herself for others, until

> "On the resurrection morn
> Soul and body meet again;
> No more sorrow, no more weeping,
> No more pain!"

One pathetic figure stood out from amidst the crowd in that churchyard—a frail old man, who in the trenches of Sebastopol had been more than once wounded, had lost one eye, and had lain for three months in the hospital at Scutari. He remembered well "the lady with the lamp."

' Every night she always came through the hospital with a lamp when the medical officers had left us. We tried to keep awake so that we should see her. Take me to pray at her graveside that Heaven reward her." And so they brought him.

Though by her own wish she was thus laid beside her father and mother in the quiet village churchyard, the great heart of London throbbed with its weight of loving gratitude for the gentle woman who had come forward and stood so bravely in the breach when war and pestilence were mowing down England's soldiers, and who since then by precept and example had raised up an army of women to follow in her footsteps, to heal the wounds inflicted by men's passions, to nurse the sick, to comfort the dying. The lamp she lit was verily the lamp of knowledge. No idle fantasy, no sentimental feelings had place in her code; work, love, and knowledge were what she called for in those who would follow in her wake. She possessed every quality needful for the great position she was called upon to occupy in the world's history—courage, single-mindedness, and a capacity for organisation and command rarely to be found united in one individual woman. She stands forth, and ever will stand forth, the pattern of a noble, gracious woman, full of pity and tenderness, as all good women are, with strength and knowledge to cope with all the difficulties of a position, until then unknown, and which was of her own creating—the fruit of years of steady preparation. So she has passed away, but not out of the memory of man, for her work remains indelible, and daily, nay hourly, from sick and dying beds, thankful hearts arise and call her blessed.

And from the dome of St. Paul's the summons came, calling the citizens of London to join in prayer, praise, and thanksgiving to God, who had sent such a woman into the world for our example as she whom, her work on earth being finished, He had now called back to Himself.

And a great multitude answered to the call. Nurses—her children—climbed the steps of the great cathedral, soldiers and civilians, old and young, all bent on doing honour to her who had just passed out of their midst and yet was still amongst them.

There are those who never die in the memory of men, and surely Florence Nightingale was one of these. In an unedited poem of Sir Edwin Arnold's, written in his boyhood, this comes home to us in the beauty of her name—birds and flowers:

> "'Tis good that thy name springs
> From two of earth's fairest things
> A stately city and a sweet-voiced bird.
> 'Tis well that in all homes,
> Where thy kind story comes,
> And brave eyes fill, that pleasant sounds be heard.
> Oh voice! in night of fear
> Like night's birds sweet to hear,
> Oh strong heart! set like city on a hill:
> Ah watcher! worn and pale;
> Dear Florence Nightingale,
> We give thee thanks for thy good work and will."